Rad Tech's Guide to
MRI: Basic Physics, Instrumentation, and Quality Control

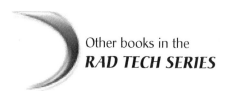

Other books in the
RAD TECH SERIES

Rad Tech's Guide to
MRI: Basic Physics, Instrumentation, and Quality Control

William Faulkner, BS, RT(R), (MR), (CT)

Director of Education, Chattanooga Imaging
President, William Faulkner & Associates
Vice-President, OutSource, Inc.
Chattanooga, Tennessee

Series Editor
Euclid Seeram, RTR, BSc, MSc, FCAMRT
Medical Imaging Advanced Studies
British Columbia Institute of Technology
Burnaby, British Columbia, Canada

b
**Blackwell
Science**

©2002 by Blackwell Science, Inc.

EDITORIAL OFFICES:
Commerce Place, 350 Main Street, Malden, Massachusetts 02148, USA
Osney Mead, Oxford OX2 0EL, England
25 John Street, London WC1N 2BS, England
23 Ainslie Place, Edinburgh EH3 6AJ, Scotland
54 University Street, Carlton, Victoria 3053, Australia

OTHER EDITORIAL OFFICES:
Blackwell Wissenschafts-Verlag GmbH, Kurfürstendamm 57, 10707 Berlin, Germany
Blackwell Science KK, MG Kodenmacho Building, 7-10 Kodenmacho Nihombashi,
    Chuo-ku, Tokyo 104, Japan
Iowa State University Press, A Blackwell Science Company, 2121 S. State Avenue,
    Ames, Iowa 50014-8300, USA

DISTRIBUTORS:

The Americas
  Blackwell Publishing
  c/o AIDC
  P.O. Box 20
  50 Winter Sport Lane
  Williston, VT 05495-0020
  (Telephone orders: 800-216-2522;
      fax orders: 802-864-7626)
Australia
  Blackwell Science Pty, Ltd.
  54 University Street
  Carlton, Victoria 3053
  (Telephone orders: 03-9347-0300;
      fax orders: 03-9349-3016)

Outside The Americas and Australia
  Blackwell Science, Ltd.
  c/o Marston Book Services, Ltd.
  P.O. Box 269
  Abingdon
  Oxon OX14 4YN
  England
  (Telephone orders: 44-01235-465500;
      fax orders: 44-01235-465555)

Acquisitions: Beverly Copland
Development: Julia Casson
Production: GraphCom Corporation
Manufacturing: Lisa Flanagan
Marketing Manager: Toni Fournier
Cover and interior design: Dana Peick, GraphCom Corporation
Typesetting: GraphCom Corporation
Printed and bound by Sheridan Books, Inc., USA
Printed in the United States of America
First Published 2002

5   2006

The Blackwell Science logo is a trade mark of Blackwell Science Ltd., registered at the United Kingdom Trade Marks Registry.

      Library of Congress Cataloging-in-Publication Data

Faulkner, William (William H.)
    Rad tech's guide to MRI : basic physics, instrumentation, and quality control /
  by William Faulkner.
        p. ; cm.—(Rad tech's guide series)
    ISBN 13: 978-0-632-04505-1
    ISBN 10: 0-632-04505-1
    1. Magnetic resonance imaging. 2. Nuclear magnetic resonance. 3.Radiologic
technologists.
    [DNLM: 1. Magnetic Resonance Imaging—methods—Examination Questions.
    2. Magnetic Resonance Imaging—methods—Handbooks. 3. Magnetic
Resonance Imaging—instrumentation—Examination Questions. 4. Magnetic
Resonance Imaging—instrumentation—Handbooks. 5. Quality Control—
Examination Questions. 6. Quality Control—Handbooks. WN 39 F263r 2001]
    I. Title. II. Series.
RC78.7.N83 F385 2001
616.07'548—dc21

                                                                    2001001709

For Tricia and Amber

Notice: The indications and dosages of all drugs in this book have been recommended in the medical literature and conform to the practices of the general community. The medications described and treatment prescriptions suggested do not necessarily have specific approval by the Food and Drug Administration for use in the diseases and dosages for which they are recommended. The package insert for each drug should be consulted for use and dosage as approved by the FDA. Because standards for usage change, it is advisable to keep abreast of revised recommendations, particularly those concerning new drugs.

TABLE OF CONTENTS

SERIES EDITOR'S FOREWORD

Blackwell Science's Rad Tech Series in radiologic technology is intended to provide a clear and comprehensive coverage of a wide range of topics and prepare students to write their entry-to-practice registration examination. Additionally, this series can be used by working technologists to review essential and practical concepts and principles and to use them as tools to enhance their daily skills during the examination of patients in the radiology department.

The Rad Tech Series features short books covering the fundamental core curriculum topics for radiologic technologists at both the diploma and the specialty levels, as well as act as knowledge sources for continuing education as defined by the American Registry for Radiologic Technologists (ARRT).

The entry-to-practice series includes books on radiologic physics, equipment operation, patient care, radiographic technique, radiologic procedures, radiation protection, image production and evaluation, and quality control. This specialty series features books on computed tomography (CT)—physics and instrumentation, patient care and safety, and imaging procedures; mammography; and quality management in imaging sciences.

In *Rad Tech's Guide to MRI: Basic Physics, Instrumentation, and Quality Control*, Bill Faulkner, a renowned educator MRI, presents a clear and concise coverage on the physics and instrumentation of MRI. Topics include fundamental physics, equipment components, data acquisition and processing, and image quality and artifacts, as well as flow imaging issues of primary significance to quality MRI.

Bill Faulkner has done an excellent job in explaining significant concepts that are mandatory to the successful performance of quality magnetic resonance imaging in clinical practice. Students, technologists, and educators alike will find this book a worthwhile addition to their libraries.

Enjoy the pages that follow; remember, your patients will benefit from your wisdom.

Euclid Seeram, RTR, BSc, MSc, FCAMRT
Series Editor
British Columbia, Canada

PREFACE

Rad Tech's Guide to MRI: Basic Physics, Instrumentation, and Quality Control is primarily written for those MR technologists who are reviewing for the ARRT Advanced Certification Examination in MRI. It is written from my MR lecture notes and is designed to provide a capsulated overview of the basic MRI principles. Some may think the text is oversimplified, but I believe it will provide a good foundation on which further study and reading can build. Although technology changes, the basic underlying principles do not, and I have found that having a solid understanding of the basic concepts provides the ability to assimilate newer techniques more easily.

Rad Tech's Guide to MRI: Basic Physics, Instrumentation, and Quality Control may also be used as a quick reference guide to the basic principles by those technologists new to MR.

I hope you enjoy this book, and I trust it provides assistance to you in making your career in MR rewarding.

Bill Faulkner

ACKNOWLEDGMENTS

I would like to thank all the technologists and radiologists with whom I've had the pleasure of working over the past 15 years. Their support, encouragement, and friendship have been my greatest assets. In particular, I'd like to thank my business partner, Candi Roth, for her support and guidance, both of which have been truly invaluable.

—WHF

CHAPTER 1

Hardware Overview

Chapter at a glance

INSTRUMENTATION: MAGNETS

To obtain a magnetic resonance (MR) signal from tissues, a large static magnetic field is required. The primary purpose of the static magnetic field (known as the B_0 field) is to magnetize the tissue. Recent innovations in magnet design and construction have produced some interesting and exciting improvements. Generally, the *style* of magnet employed can be described as either a vertical field (occasionally referred to as an *open MRI*) or the conventional horizontal field magnet. Regardless of the style or type of magnet used, the B_0 field must be stable and homogeneous, particularly in the central area of the magnet (isocenter) where imaging takes place.

- The vertical field magnet design uses two magnets, one above the patient and one below the patient.
- The frame, which supports the magnets, also serves to "return" the magnetic field.
- Vertical magnets generally have a reduced fringe field compared with conventional horizontal field magnets.

- The "open design" of these systems is often marketed as being less confining to the patient who is anxious or claustrophobic.
- The radio-frequency (RF) coils and gradient coils (discussed in more detail later) are flat coils located on the "face" of the magnets.
- The *receiver* or surface coils used with vertical field magnets are solenoid in design.
- Field strength and homogeneity can be increased by reducing the gap between the two magnets. The disadvantage to reducing the gap is the obvious reduction in patient area.

Regardless of whether the field is vertical or horizontal, there are three primary types of magnets: permanent, resistive, and superconducting.

Permanent Magnets

- Lower field vertical field systems historically used permanent magnets.
- Permanent magnets consist of blocks or slabs of naturally occurring ferrous material.
- Increasing the amount of material used increases the field strength, in addition to size and weight.
- Permanent magnets generally have field strengths of 0.06 to 0.35 Tesla.
- Vertical field permanent magnets generally have a relatively small fringe field.
- Because of the small fringe field, permanent magnets are often easy to sight, though their weight can be an issue.
- Permanent magnets are sensitive to the ambient room temperature.
- Changes in scan room temperature can cause the field strength to vary several gauss per degree.
- Because changes in field strength result in changes in resonant frequency, scanning may not be possible if the field drifts significantly.

Resistive Magnets

- Resistive magnets can be used in either a vertical or horizontal field system.

- Resistive magnets generally have field strengths up to 0.3 Tesla.
- Whenever electrical current is applied to a wire, a magnetic field is induced around the wire.
- To produce a static field (i.e., not alternating), direct current is required.
- Increasing the amount of current or turns of wire increases the field strength and heats the wire.
- Resistive magnets require a constant current to maintain the static field.
- Cooling of the coils is also required since the by-product of electrical resistance is heat.
- Resistive magnets can be turned off when not in use (permanent and superconductive magnets cannot be turned off).
- The earliest types of magnets used in MRI were resistive.
- Resistive magnets can also be temperature-sensitive.
- A hybrid design can use some permanent material with resistive coils.

Superconductive Magnets

- Superconductive magnets are similar to resistive magnets because they use direct current actively applied to a coil of wire to produce the static magnetic field.
- The main difference is that the coils are immersed in liquid helium (cryogen) to remove the resistance.
- Without the resistance, the electrical current can flow within a closed circuit without external power being applied.
- The flow of electrical current without resistance is known superconductivity.
- Most superconductive magnets are solenoid in design and thus exhibit a horizontal magnetic field.
- Recent innovations in magnet design allow for vertical field systems using superconducting magnets.
- Superconductive magnets are capable of achieving high field strengths.
- Small bore horizontal magnets used to image small animals and tissue samples can have field strengths of 10 Tesla or higher.

■ Superconductive magnets used in clinical MRI in the United States are currently limited by the U.S. Food and Drug Administration (FDA) to 4.0 Tesla.

■ The majority of superconductive magnets currently in clinical use range between 0.5 and 1.5 Tesla.

■ Higher field strengths produce greater fringe fields.

■ To limit or reduce the fringe field for siting purposes, magnetic shielding is employed.

■ Passive magnetic shielding uses metal in the scan room walls to confine the fringe field.

■ Active magnetic shielding uses additional coils within or around the magnet with current applied to restrain the fringe field.

■ The liquid helium used to cool the magnet coils "boils off" at various rates depending on magnet design and therefore needs to be replaced periodically.

■ Liquid helium exists at only 4° C and under great pressure. If the temperature within the vessel containing the magnet coils and liquid helium rise only slightly, then the liquid helium will boil and therefore expand at a ratio of 760:1.

■ The resultant helium gas will burst through a pressure-sensitive containment system and should vent outside the scan room through a duct system attached to the magnet.

■ In the absence of the supercooled environment, the current in the magnet coils will experience resistance, and the static field will be lost.

■ This sudden and violent loss of superconductivity is referred to as a *quench*.

■ The major advantage of superconducting technology is high field strength, which results in inherently high signal-to-noise ratio (SNR).

■ The high SNR can be "traded" for rapid scan times and increased spatial resolution.

■ The major disadvantage of superconducting technology is the high cost associated with acquisition, siting, and maintenance.

B_0 Homogeneity

Regardless of the type or style of magnet used for an MR system, the magnetic field must be as homogeneous as possible. This characteristic is particularly critical within the central area of the magnet (isocenter) where imaging takes place. The homogeneity is maximized through a process know as *shimming*. Shimming can be accomplished either *actively, passively,* or through a combination of both.

- Active shimming implies the use of additional coils within the magnet vessel or structure.
- Current applied in the shim coils either adds or subtracts from the static magnetic field to produce a field that is as homogeneous as possible.
- Passive shimming implies the use of small bits of ferrous material.
- In the case of a horizontal field magnet, the ferrous material is placed around the bore.
- In the case of a vertical field system, the material is placed on the face of the main magnets.

INSTRUMENTATION: RADIO-FREQUENCY SUBSYSTEM

Transmit

- The primary purpose of the RF subsystem is to transmit the RF pulses or field (known as the B1 field) and to receive the MR signal from tissue being examined.
- The B1 field is used to provide the necessary energy to cause the net magnetization of the tissues to tip and rotate through the transverse plane where the receiving coils are located.
- The RF subsystem consists of coils that transmit or receive the RF signals and the electronics that power them.
- Most RF subsystems in use today are digital rather than analog.
- Digital RF systems provide for finer control of the RF pulses produced in the MRI process.
- RF coils can be designed to transmit only, receive only, or transmit and receive. The decision as to what design

will be used is largely determined by the manufacturer or the overall MR system design.

- In superconducting, horizontal field systems, a large *body coil* is located within the magnet enclosure. In general, the body coil operates as a transmit-and-receive (T/R) coil.

- Body coils are used to acquire information over a large field-of-view (FOV).

- The primary disadvantage of a body coil is an inherently low SNR.

- Generally, a larger coil will produce a lower SNR. Conversely, a smaller coil will produce a higher SNR.

- To increase the SNR, smaller surface (local) coils can be placed over or around the region of interest.

- Local coils can be either a T/R coil or a receive-only coil, again, largely based on the manufacturer's preference.

- If the local coil is a receive-only coil, then the body coil transmits RF.

- Reducing the size of the local coil increases the SNR, but the area of coverage is reduced.

Local (Surface) Coils

The primary purpose of local coils is to increase the SNR. The main difficulty is to do so without excessive restriction of coverage of the area of interest. As mentioned, as the coil size is increased, the SNR is reduced. Currently, there are three main categories or types of local coils: linear, quadrature, and phased-array coils.

- The first types of local coils used in MRI were linear in design.

- Quadrature designs use additional loops and circuitry to improve the efficiency with which the MR signal is induced in the coil.

- Typically, quadrature coils produce an increase in the SNR of approximately 40% compared with a linear coil of the same size.

- Vertical field magnets require the use of solenoid coils because of the orientation of B_0. Generally, the solenoid configuration is more efficient compared with a liner coil of similar size.

- It is possible to combine coils electronically to improve signal uniformity through a region of interest.
- When two coils are combined in a manner such that they use the same receiver electronics, this is referred to as a *Helmholtz pair.*
- The Helmholtz pair has been used in coils designed to image the cervical spine, neck, and bilateral temporo-mandibular joints.
- Although a Helmholtz pair can improve the signal homogeneity across a region of interest, the SNR is not necessarily increased, which is a result primarily of coupling between the coils.
- Phased-array coils allow for increased area of coverage without a reduction in the SNR.
- Typically, a phased-array coil consists of an array of coils designed to cover a particular area of the anatomy such as the spine, abdomen, or extremities.
- The major distinguishing characteristic of phased-array coil is that each active coil in the array is connected to its own receiver.
- Multiple receivers contribute to the increased cost of phased-array technology.
- With phased-array coils, one realizes the coverage of the entire array, but the SNR characteristic of each coil within the array.
- RF coils must be "tuned" for the specific Larmor frequency of the MR system for which they are designed and cannot be used on systems operating at a different field strength.
- Generally, the tuning is set by the manufacturer and cannot be changed on site.

INSTRUMENTATION: GRADIENT SUBSYSTEM

The primary purpose of the gradient subsystem is to select the slice and imaging plane and to spatially encode the MR signal spatially. A gradient subsystem consists of coils and the electronics that power them. The term gradient means slope or incline. A gradient magnetic field is therefore one that varies in intensity over distance. During the *imaging* process, gradient magnetic fields are also varied over time.

- Gradient magnetic fields are superimposed over the primary magnetic field.
- Gradient magnetic fields are produced by applying current to the gradient coils.
- There are three sets of gradient coils in MR systems.
- The coil that is used to vary the intensity of the magnetic field in the head-to-foot direction is referred to as a z *gradient coil.*
- The coil that is used to vary the intensity of the magnetic field in the right-to-left direction is referred to as an x *gradient coil.*
- The coil that is used to vary the intensity of the magnetic field in the anterior-to-posterior direction is referred to as a y *gradient coil.*
- The term *amplitude* refers to the severity of the slope of the gradient magnetic field.
- A high-amplitude gradient will have a steep slope and will therefore greatly vary the intensity of the magnetic field in a given direction.
- *Polarity* (either positive or negative) refers to whether the gradient magnetic field is creating a field greater than or less than the frequency of B_0.
- The maximal amplitude of gradient magnetic fields is described in units of millitesla per meter (mT/m).
- Currently, most MR systems have gradient subsystems capable of achieving maximal amplitudes of 15 mT/m or greater.
- Higher gradient amplitudes offer the benefits of thinner slices and smaller FOVs.
- The speed at which a gradient magnetic field attains its maximal amplitude is identified by its *rise time.*
- Rise time is expressed in units of microseconds (μsec).
- Currently, typical rise times range from 500 to approximately 120 μsec.
- Another way to express gradient performance is *slew rate.*
- Slew rate refers to the acceleration of the gradient magnetic field to its maximal amplitude.
- Slew rate is expressed in units of Tesla/meter/second (T/m/sec).

- Currently, typical slew rates for gradient systems range from approximately 10 to over 100 T/m/sec.
- Increased slew rates offer the benefit of reduced echo times (TE), increased number of slices per repetition times (TR), shorter TR for three-dimensional (3-D) sequences, and improved image quality with echo planar and fast spin echo sequences.

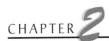

Fundamental Principles

Chapter at a glance

ELECTROMAGNETISM: FARADAY'S LAW OF INDUCTION

Electricity and magnetism go hand-in-hand. Whenever an electrical current is produced in a wire, a magnetic field is produced around the wire. As the current in the wire increases, the magnetic field increases. This characteristic is the basic principle behind the construction of resistive and super-conductive magnets discussed in Chapter 1. Magnets or magnetic fields can also be used to induce electrical current in conductors. This principle is known as *Faraday's Law of Induction* and is written as $\Delta B/\Delta t = \Delta V$ Faraday's Law of Induction states that moving a magnet or changing a magnetic field (ΔB) over time (Δt) in the presence of a conductor will induce a voltage (ΔV) in the conductor. As the magnetic field moving through the conductor is increased, the current induced in the conductor is increased. As the time decreases (shortens)—in other words, the more rapid the change in the magnetic field—the induced current is increased. Faraday's Law of Induction is the basic principle by which MR signals are detected.

Magnetism

Magnetic Properties of Matter

All matter has magnetic properties. There are three types of magnetic properties: diamagnetic, paramagnetic, and ferromagnetic.

- Diamagnetic substances exhibit a slight negative or repelling effect when placed in an externally applied magnetic field.
- Diamagnetic substances are said to have a − 1 susceptibility.
- The diamagnetic effect is weak.
- Gold is an example of a diamagnetic substance.
- Paramagnetic substances exhibit a slight increase in their magnetic field when placed in an externally applied magnetic field.
- Paramagnetic substances are said to have a + 1 susceptibility.
- Gadolinium is an example of a paramagnetic substance.
- The paramagnetic properties of gadolinium make it an excellent contrast agent for magnetic resonance imaging.
- Some substances have both diamagnetic and paramagnetic properties. In this event, since the paramagnetic effects are stronger, the substance exhibits paramagnetic characteristics.
- Ferromagnetic substances are similar to paramagnetic substances in that they become magnetized when placed in an externally applied magnetic field.
- Ferromagnetic substances, however, will remain magnetized when the externally applied field is removed.
- Iron is an example of a ferromagnetic substance.
- A dipole is a magnet with two poles: north and south.
- By convention, the magnetic field of a dipole runs from the north pole around to the south pole.
- When two identical poles are brought together, the resultant fields oppose each other and thus they repel.
- When two opposite poles are brought together, the resultant fields add and the two magnets are pulled toward each other.
- The strength of a magnetic field is expressed in terms of Gauss or Tesla.

- Gauss is the smaller unit of measure compared with Tesla.
- The earth's magnetic field strength is approximately 0.5 Gauss.
- One Tesla equals 10,000 Gauss.

Nuclear Magnetism

In the early days of magnetic resonance imaging, the term *nuclear magnetic resonance* (NMR) was used. The word *nuclear*, however, elicited visions of radioactivity, thus the name was changed to *magnetic resonance imaging* (MRI). In reality, the term *nuclear* as it is used in NMR refers to the nucleus of the atom. Certain nuclei have properties that cause them to display magnetic characteristics. Of all the magnetically active nuclei, hydrogen is the most abundant in the human body and is therefore used in clinical MRI.

- The hydrogen atom consists of a single proton.
- The proton has mass, a positive charge, and spins on its axis.
- The spinning motion of a positively charged particle results in a magnetic field around the proton.
- The proton's magnetic field is often termed the *magnetic moment*.
- For this reason, hydrogen is considered *magnetically active*.
- Other nuclei (e.g., carbon, phosphorus, sodium) are also magnetically active because of their nuclear makeup.
- Hydrogen, however, is nearly 100% abundant in the human body and has a relatively large magnetic moment.
- In the human body, hydrogen exists essentially in only two molecules: water and fat.
- For these reasons, hydrogen is ideal for use in MRI.

BEHAVIOR OF HYDROGEN IN A MAGNETIC FIELD

Because the hydrogen proton, or *spin*, has a magnetic moment, it exhibits certain behavior when placed in a large, externally applied magnetic field (B_0).

Alignment and Net Magnetization

- Within seconds of tissue being placed in a magnetic field, the hydrogen protons will assume one of two possible spin states or energy levels: high-energy or low-energy.

- One way to explain the spin states is to refer to the protons as aligning with or against the external magnetic field.
- Spins aligned parallel (i.e., with the direction of B_0) are in the low-energy state.
- Spins aligned antiparallel (i.e., against the direction of B_0) are in the high-energy state.
- At any given time, there will be a slight majority of spins in the low-energy state (parallel).
- The magnetic moments of spins in the high-energy state cancel the effect of an equal number of spins in the low-energy state.
- Since there is a greater number of spins in the low-energy state compared with the high-energy state, the magnetic moments of these spins, in the so-called *spin excess*, add to form a magnetic field referred to as the *net magnetization vector* (NMV).
- The NMV is therefore aligned parallel to B_0 (external static magnetic field).
- The previous text describes a condition known as *thermal equilibrium*.
- The energy delta between the two spin states is field-strength dependent.
- The energy delta between the two spin states is directly proportional to B_0.
- Although there is always a greater number of spins aligned parallel versus antiparallel, at higher field strengths, there is a greater number when compared with lower field strengths.
- For this reason, the tissue magnetization (i.e., NMV) is greater at higher field strengths.

Precession

- The hydrogen protons also precess around the axis of the static magnetic field.
- The precession motion of the proton is often compared with the motion of a spinning top or gyroscope.
- The spinning gyroscope exerts a force (spin angular momentum) perpendicular to the direction of the spin.

- Gravity pulls downward causing the gyroscope to wobble or precess.
- With the hydrogen proton, the spinning motion of the proton produces spin angular momentum in the same fashion.
- Additionally, the proton exhibits a magnetic field (magnetic moment).
- The ratio of the spin angular momentum of the proton to its magnetic moment is known as the *gyromagnetic ratio*.
- The gyromagnetic ratio varies with each magnetically active nucleus and is expressed in units of megahertz/Tesla (MHz/T).
- The gyromagnetic ratio for hydrogen is 42.56 MHz/T.
- The actual precessional frequency for hydrogen can be calculated from the Larmor equation (Figure 2-1).
- Increasing B_0 causes the precessional or resonant frequency of hydrogen to increase. Decreasing B_0 causes the resonant frequency to decrease.
- The frequency at which the hydrogen protons precess is known as the *Larmor frequency* or *resonant frequency*.

A little more about thermal equilibrium:

- At thermal equilibrium, the hydrogen spins do not precess at exactly the same frequency.
- Several factors contribute to their lack of phase coherence. Primarily, hydrogen spins are inhomogeneities and have chemical shift effects.
- Inhomogeneities in the magnetic field are always present. Although the magnet is *shimmed*, when a patient is placed in the magnet, the field is distorted.
- Inhomogeneities also occur within the body, which are known as *local field inhomogeneities*.

$$\omega_0 = B_0 \cdot \gamma$$

$$1.5 \text{ T} \times 42.6 \text{ MHz/T} = 63.9 \text{ MHz}$$

$$0.2 \text{ T} \times 42.6 \text{ MHz/T} = 8.52 \text{ MHz}$$

Figure 2-1 The effect of field strength on the precessional frequency is shown. As the field strength increases, the processional frequency increases.

- Local inhomogeneities can be caused by metal or foreign materials in the body, as well as by areas with vastly different magnetic properties.

- When metal is present within the body, the magnetic field around the metal is greatly distorted.

- This distortion causes the resonant frequencies of the spins to vary greatly.

- Smaller distortions are observed at air-tissue interfaces. Although these distortions cause a variance in the spin's resonant frequencies, the amount of variance (i.e., dephasing) is not as great compared with the presence of metal objects or implants.

- The molecular environment can also affect the phase coherence among the spins.

- A water molecule consists of oxygen and hydrogen. The oxygen atom "steals" the hydrogen's electron. As a result, the hydrogen proton "experiences" the external magnetic field without the normal presence of its orbital electron.

- A fat molecule consists of carbon and hydrogen. The carbon atom does not alter the orbit of the hydrogen's electron. As a result, the hydrogen proton "experiences" the external field with its orbital electron in place.

- The presence or absence of the orbital electron causes the proton in a water molecule to "see" a slightly higher field than the proton in a fat molecule.

- Hydrogen in water will therefore precess slightly faster than hydrogen in fat.

- This difference in precessional frequency is known as *chemical shift*.

- The amount of chemical shift (i.e., frequency difference) is field-strength dependent, expressed as 3.5 parts per million (ppm).

- For example, at 1.5 Tesla, 1 ppm = 63.86 Hz. Therefore 3.5 ppm = 224 Hz, which means that hydrogen in water will precess 224 Hz faster than the hydrogen in fat.

- The effect of local field inhomogeneities and chemical shift causes the spins to precess out of phase at thermal equilibrium.

CHAPTER 3

Production of Magnetic Resonance Signal

The magnetic resonance (MR) signal is induced in a receiver coil when the net magnetization vector (NMV) is rotated through the coil. This chapter will examine how this process is accomplished.

- Radio-frequency (RF) energy is nonionizing, electromagnetic radiation.
- A radio wave is an oscillating electromagnetic field.
- Exposing magnetized tissue to an RF field at the Larmor frequency (dictated by the strength of B_0), first causes the hydrogen spins to begin precessing *in phase*, which causes the NMV to precess as well.
- As the RF pulse continues, some of the spins in the low-energy state absorb energy from the RF field and move to the high-energy state.
- As more and more spins absorb energy, changing spin states, the NMV begins to tip outward, away from the longitudinal or z axis.
- When the spins are evenly distributed between the two spin states, the NMV will now be precessing through the xy (transverse) plane, 90 degrees away from its original orientation in the z axis (Figure 3-1).
- Tipping the NMV 90 degrees away from the z axis is referred to as applying a 90-degree flip angle.
- Another way to phrase the effects of applying a 90-degree flip angle is to say that the longitudinal magnetization (Mz) is converted to transverse magnetization (Mxy).
- Increasing the amount of RF energy will cause an increase in the flip angle.
- To double the flip angle, a four-fold increase in RF power is required.

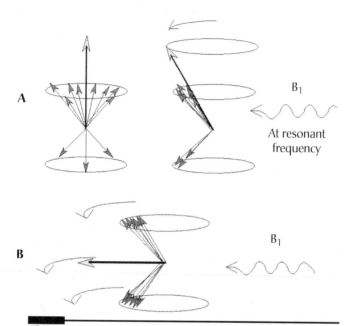

Figure 3-1 The effect of applying a radio-frequency pulse at the resonant or Larmor frequency is demonstrated. *A,* The spins begin to precess in phase. As a result, the net magnetization vector also precesses. *B,* As the pulse continues, some of the spins in the low-energy state gain energy from the radio-frequency pulse and move to the high-energy state, which causes net magnetization vector to tip outward and to precess through the transverse (xy) plane.

- The amount of power necessary to achieve a desired flip angle will depend on several factors, including the field strength and the type of RF coil used for transmitting the RF signal and is determined during *prescan* or "tuning" performed before each scan.
- When the desired flip angle is achieved, the RF pulse is discontinued to allow for detection of the signal.
- As the NMV is precessing through the xy plane, it will precess through a receiver coil oriented in the same plane (Figure 3-2).
- In accordance with Faraday's Law of Induction, an MR signal will be induced in the coil.

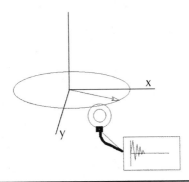

Figure 3-2 As the NMV is precessing through the xy plane, it will precess through a receiver coil, which is oriented in the same plane.

- The signal induced in a receiver coil immediately following an RF excitation pulse is known as the *free induction decay* (FID).
- The FID decays rapidly after removal of the RF pulse (see Figure 3-2).
- The FID is a result of the shrinking of the NMV as it rotates through the xy plane.
- The NMV shrinks because spins rapidly loose phase coherence after the RF pulse has been removed.
- Simultaneously but independently, some of the spins in the high-energy state lose energy gained from the RF pulse and return to the low-energy state.
- As more spins return to the low-energy state, the NMV again increases in z axis.

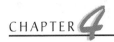

Relaxation

Following excitation by the radio-frequency (RF) pulse, the spins relax toward equilibrium. This relaxation occurs through two simultaneous yet independent processes: T1 and T2. T2 relaxation refers to the loss of magnetization in the transverse (xy) plane. T1 is the recovery of magnetization along the z axis.

- As mentioned, following removal of the RF pulse, the spins immediately and rapidly loose phase coherence.

- T2 (spin-spin relaxation) is caused by an exchange of energy among the spins, which results in dephasing.

- Inhomogeneities in the field and within the tissues further results in dephasing.

- Additionally, hydrogen in fat and water molecules precesses at different frequencies.

- This difference in precessional frequency from the chemical-molecular environment is known as *chemical shift*.

- Chemical shift is field-strength dependent and is expressed as a constant of 3.5 ppm.

- The combination of T2 (spin-spin interaction), inhomogeneities, and chemical shift results in a rapid loss of transverse magnetization, known as T2* (pronounced T2 star).

- The FID therefore decays at a rate based on T2*.

- Simultaneously but independently, the longitudinal magnetization again increases along the z axis as spins in the high-energy state loose energy.

- The rate at which the longitudinal magnetization increases is known as the tissue's *T1 time*.

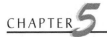

Tissue Characteristics

Chapter at a glance

Several intrinsic magnetic resonance (MR) properties of tissues contribute to image contrast, including T1 and T2 relaxation times, spin (proton) density, and flow motion. The properties are based on the molecular makeup of the tissues. Tissues in the body consist primarily of fat and water. For this reason, these molecules will be the primary focus of this text.

PROTON DENSITY

- Spin density is simply a representation of the number of hydrogen protons (spins) in a given volume of tissue.
- In the human body, cerebral spinal fluid (CSF) has the highest spin density.
- Spin density is usually expressed as a percentage value, with CSF being 100%.
- Other tissues have lower spin densities but do not differ greatly.
- The only exceptions, as examples, are air and cortical bone. Because of their extremely low spin density, air and cortical bone produce essentially no MR signal and are observed as signal voids on MR images.

T2 RELAXATION

- T2 relaxation refers to the loss or decay of transverse magnetization.

- The decay occurs exponentially and is defined as the time required for 63% of the tissue's transverse magnetization to decay.
- The primary mechanism of T2 decay is an exchange of energy among the spins.
- As the spins swap energy states (energy exchange), they *dephase*.
- Because of the interaction among the spins, T2 relaxation is also referred to as *spin-spin relaxation*.
- Dephasing of transverse magnetization from T2 cannot be reversed or corrected.
- Fat has a short or rapid T2 decay, and water has a long T2 decay.
- T2 times of tissues are usually measured in milliseconds (msec).

T1 Relaxation

- T1 relaxation refers to the recovery of magnetization along the longitudinal or z axis.
- The recovery occurs exponentially and is defined as the time required for 63% of the tissue's longitudinal magnetization to recover.
- The primary mechanism of T1 recovery is the loss of the spins' energy to the surrounding molecular lattice.
- For this reason, T1 recovery is also known as *spin-lattice relaxation*.
- Fat has a short or rapid T1 recovery, and water has a long T1 recovery.
- T1 times of tissues are typically measured in seconds
- A tissue's T1 recovery time is also affected by temperature and field strength.
- Increasing the tissue's temperature lengthens its T1 recovery time.
- Reducing the external field strength (B_0) shortens its T1 recovery time.

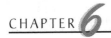

Data Acquisition and Image Formation

Chapter at a glance

PULSE SEQUENCES

A pulse sequence, as the name implies, is a series of radio-frequency (RF) pulses. Control of the image contrast is accomplished by controlling the timing of the RF pulses in the pulse sequence, as well as by selecting the type of pulse sequence. The two primary types of pulse sequences are spin echo and gradient echo.

Spin Echo

- A spin echo pulse sequence begins with a 90-degree RF pulse followed by a 180-degree RF pulse.

- As previously discussed, the purpose of the 90-degree pulse is to convert the longitudinal magnetization to transverse magnetization.

- After the RF pulse is removed, the spins begin to rapidly dephase at a rate that is dependent on T2* (free induction decay [FID]).

- After a specified time, a 180-degree RF pulse is applied (Figure 6-1).

- The purpose of the 180-degree RF pulse is to "flip" the magnetization through the transverse plane and refocus the spins that have dephased as a result of slight field inhomogeneities and chemical shifts.

- As the spins refocus, or rephase, the MR signal increases but then decreases once again as the spins dephase in the other "direction".

- The classic analogy is that of runners in a race. As the race begins, the faster runners get in front of the slower runners. If, at a specified point, the runners were to turn 180 degrees, the faster runners will be behind the slower runners. As they return towards the starting line, the faster runners will catch the slower runners and they will all be *in phase* as they met. As they continued, however, the faster runners will once again get ahead of the slower runners.

- In a magnetic resonance (MR) pulse sequence, the operator can choose the time between the 90-degree pulse

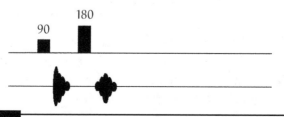

Figure 6-1 A simplified spin echo pulse sequence diagram.

and the formation of the echo. This parameter is known as the time to the echo (TE), usually expressed in milli-seconds (msec).

- One millisecond is equal to 1/1000 of a second.
- The 180-degree RF pulse is applied at a time equal to one half of the TE selected by the operator. For example, if the operator selects a 20 msec TE, the 180-degree pulse will be automatically applied 10 msec after the 90-degree pulse.
- Occasionally, the time between the 90-degree pulse and the 180-degree pulse is referred to as *tau*.
- This sequence (90-180) is repeated after a specified interval selected by the operator. This interval is known as the repetition time (TR).

Gradient Echo

- A gradient echo sequence begins with an RF pulse that may be 90 degrees but can be less when so selected by the operator. This flip angle is selected based on the image contrast desired and will be discussed in more detail later.
- The echo is formed by the application of two gradient magnetic fields. The first gradient application dephases the spins. The second application of the gradient is the opposite polarity to the dephasing lobe, producing the exact opposite magnetic field.
- Spins that sensed a reduction in the magnetic field and "slowed down" now sense an increase in the magnetic field and "speed up," refocusing the available transverse magnetization and producing an echo (Figure 6-2).

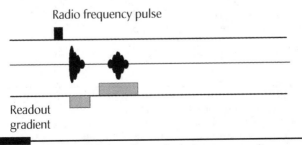

Radio frequency pulse

Readout
gradient

Figure 6-2 A simplified gradient echo pulse sequence diagram.

- As with the spin echo pulse sequence, the time between the initial or excitation pulse of the sequence and the echo is the TE.
- The time between repetitions of the sequence is the TR.

Inversion Recovery

When desired, a sequence can begin with a 180-degree inversion pulse. This type of sequence is often called *inversion recovery*. An inversion pulse can be used with either a spin echo or gradient echo sequence. The time between the 180-degree inversion pulse and the 90-degree pulse in a spin echo sequence or the initial RF pulse in a gradient echo sequence is controlled by the operator and is known as the *time of inversion* or TI (Figure 6-3).

IMAGE CONTRAST CONTROL

One of the major advantages of magnetic resonance imaging (MRI) over other types of imaging modalities is the ability to control the image contrast. Contrast observed on an MR image depends on the intrinsic properties of tissues: proton density, T1 and T2 relaxation times, as well as the extrinsic parameters under the operators control: TR, TE, TI, and flip angle.

Time to the Echo and T2

- As mentioned, in a spin echo sequence, the TE is the time between the initial 90-degree pulse and the echo.
- Because the 180-degree pulse does not correct for any loss of dephasing from spin-spin or T2 relaxation, the

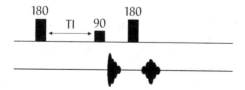

Figure 6-3 The time between the 180-degree inversion pulse and the 90-degree pulse in a spin echo sequence or the initial radio frequency pulse in a gradient echo sequence is under operator control and is known as the time of inversion.

quicker the echo is formed, the less the loss of magnetization (and therefore loss of signal) from T2 relaxation.

■ Acquiring a sequence with a longer TE will increase the amount of T2 decay that occurs between the 90-degree pulse and the echo.

■ An image acquired with an extremely short TE (e.g., 20 msec or less) will therefore have few effects from T2 decay.

■ An image acquired with a longer TE (e.g., 80 msec or higher) will therefore exhibit a greater amount of contrast from the T2 differences between tissues.

■ In this way, TE controls the amount of T2 contrast in an MR image. Reducing the TE reduces the T2 weighting in the image. Increasing the TE increases the T2 weighting in the image (Figure 6-4).

Repetition Time and T1

■ As mentioned, the TR is the time between repetitions of the pulse sequence.

■ The longer the TR selected, the greater the amount of time allowing for regrowth of the longitudinal magnetization (Mz).

■ When a short TR is selected (e.g., 400 msec), only the spins with a short T1 time (such as fat) will be given suf-

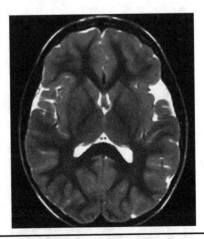

Figure 6-4 T2-weighted image.

ficient time to recover. Spins with longer T1 times (such as water or cerebrospinal fluid [CSF]) will be more saturated (i.e., they will exhibit less longitudinal recovery).

- If a longer TR is selected (e.g., 2000 msec), all spins will be given more time for longitudinal recovery to occur.
- In this way, TR controls the amount of T1 contrast in an MR image. Reducing the TR increases the T1 weighting in the image. Increasing the TR reduces the T1 weighting in the image (Figure 6-5).

Combining Repetition Time and Time to the Echo to Control Image Contrast

If an image with T1 weighting is desired, then a short TE is selected (20 msec or less). Using a short TE does not make an image T1-weighted, but rather, it makes it less T2-weighted. Selecting a short TR (600 msec or less) will then produce an image with T1 weighting. The exact TR depends on the tissues being imaged and the field strength (because T1 times are field-strength dependent). In the brain, at 1.5 Tesla, TR times of 400 msec to 500 msec are usually desired. As the TR increases, the contrast between gray and white matter will be less. At lower field strengths, 0.2 to 0.5 Tesla, lower TR times (usually 250 msec to 400 msec) are required for optimal gray-white matter contrast.

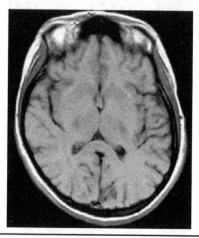

Figure 6-5 T1-weighted image.

If an image with T2 weighting is desired, then a long TR is selected (2000 msec or higher). Using a long TR does not make an image T2-weighted, but rather, it makes it less T1-weighted. Selecting a long TE (80 msec or higher) will then produce an image with T2 weighting. Increasing the TR from 2000 msec will increase the signal from CSF or water and will therefore increase the contrast between certain structures. As a general rule, in the brain and spine, TR times of 4000 msec or higher will produce images with high contrast between CSF and surrounding structures.

If proton density (PD) weighting is desired, a short TE is selected (20 msec or less) to reduce the T2 weighting. A long TR is then selected (2000 msec or higher) to reduce the T1 weighting (Figure 6-6). When acquiring PD-weighted images in the brain, generally, a TR of between 2000 and 3000 msec is selected. As mentioned, when higher TR times are selected, the signal intensity from CSF is increased. High signal from CSF may actually reduce the contrast between certain abnormalities and CSF. Multiple sclerosis (MS) plaques are a good example. MS plaques usually occur in the periventricular white matter and have a moderately high signal on PD-weighted images. If the signal intensity from CSF is too high, then the plaques may be indistinguishable from the adjacent CSF. In any event, increasing the TR will increase the signal intensity from CSF and vise versa.

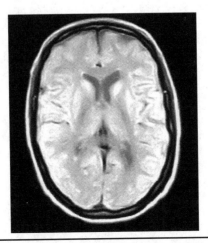

Figure 6-6 Proton density–weighted image.

Gradient Echo Contrast Control

Using gradient echo sequences, images with T2 or PD contrasts can be acquired using short TR times. The benefit of this technique is a reduction in scanning times over sequences using longer TR times. Up to this point, we have been assuming that the pulse sequence begins with a 90-degree pulse. In gradient echo sequences, the flip angle must be selected, as well as the TR and TE.

- If a short TR time is selected, then only the spins with short or rapid T1 times will be given sufficient time to recover longitudinal magnetization.
- To enable longitudinal recovery to occur with spins exhibiting long T1 times, lower flip angles are selected.
- As the flip angle is reduced (assuming constant TR), spins with longer T1 times exhibit greater longitudinal recovery, and the image becomes less T1-weighted.
- In this way, flip angle controls the T1 and PD weighting in an MR image.
- Reducing the flip angle has the same effect on image contrast as increasing the TR (i.e., the image becomes less T1-weighted).
- Increasing the flip angle has the same effect on image contrast as reducing the TR (i.e., the image becomes more T1-weighted).

Gradient Echo Sequences and T2*. As mentioned, the purpose of the 180-degree refocusing pulse in a spin echo pulse sequence is to refocus or correct for dephasing resulting from slight inhomogeneities and chemical shifts. In a gradient echo pulse sequence, the echo is formed by the reversal of a gradient magnetic field only (i.e., a 180-degree pulse is not used). Gradient echo sequences are often referred to as a gradient recalled echo (GRE) sequence. Because of the lack of the 180-degree RF pulse in a GRE sequence, the decay of transverse magnetization is a result of not only T2, but also the effects of B_0, as well as local inhomogeneities and chemical shifts. The addition of these extrinsic (environmental) effects produces a more rapid rate of transverse magnetization decay, known as T2* (Figure 6-7). Because of these differences between spin echo and gradient echo sequences, GRE sequences are often referred to as T2*.

Steady State versus Spoiled. There are two basic types of GRE sequences: steady state GRE and spoiled GRE. The selection of a steady state or spoiled sequence is based on the type of contrast desired (Figure 6-8).

- When the TR is shorter than the T1 and T2* of tissues (generally less than 250 msec), a condition known as steady state exists.
- In a steady state, residual transverse magnetization exists from one TR to the next, because the short TR time does not allow for the normal transverse decay.
- Typically, when a steady state GRE sequence is used, the signal from CSF remains bright regardless of the flip angle selected.
- To obtain T1-weighted images without the effects of the steady state (e.g., bright signal from fluid), a spoiled GRE sequence is used.

$$\frac{1}{T2} + \frac{1}{T2'} = \frac{1}{T2*}$$

Figure 6-7 T2 represents spin-spin relaxation, T2* represents the effects from inhomogeneities and chemical shift.

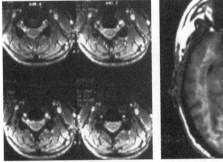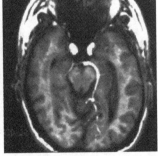

Figure 6-8 The axial cervical spine series on the left was acquired using a steady state gradient recalled echo (GRE) sequence. The axial image of the brain on the right was acquired using a spoiling GRE sequence.

- The term *spoiling* refers to the removal of the residual transverse magnetization between excitation pulses.
- Spoiling can be achieved by the use of a gradient magnetic field (gradient spoiling) or by varying the phase angle of the excitation pulse (RF spoiling).
- Using a spoiled GRE sequence, images with T1 weighting can be obtained when using short TR GRE sequences.
- Generally, when images with high signal from fluid are desired (e.g., T2* or PD weighting), a steady state sequence is selected.
- When images with T1 contrast are desired, a spoiled sequence is selected.

Inversion Recovery Contrast

Inversion recovery (IR) sequences were initially used to acquire images with strong T1 weighting. Although this application is still valid, newer uses have emerged to allow for improved tissue contrasts. Generally, inversion sequences begin with a 180-degree RF pulse to invert longitudinal magnetization (Mz). After the inversion, there is an operator-specified delay time known as the time of inversion (TI). In a spin echo inversion sequence, the initializing 180-degree RF pulse (inversion pulse) is followed by a 90-degree pulse and then a 180-degree pulse. Inversion pulses may be used with any type of pulse sequences (e.g., spin echo, GRE, echo planar images). For the purposes of the following discussion, spin echo sequence will be assumed.

- Following the application of the inversion pulse, the longitudinal magnetization will regrow along the z axis.
- If the 90-degree pulse is applied when a given tissue's magnetization has regrown to the zero or null point (i.e., neither negative nor positive), then the signal from the tissue will be null.
- As a rule, when a TI is selected that is 69% of a tissue's T1 time, the signal from the tissue will be zero (assuming a TR of sufficient length to allow for full longitudinal recovery).
- Therefore the TI is selected based on the desired tissue contrast.

- An inversion sequence that uses a short TI such that fat is nulled is often referred to as STIR (short TI recovery).
- STIR sequences are useful in musculoskeletal examinations. In the presence of bone marrow diseases, normal bone marrow, which has a high fat content, will appear as a hypointense signal relative to diseases, which has a high fluid content (Figure 6-9).
- In the brain, most diseased tissues are associated with an increase in fluid.
- Using the standard, long TR and long TE spin echo sequence, the technologist is often unable to separate the high signal from pathologic fluid from the signal of CSF.
- A fluid attenuated inversion recovery (FLAIR) sequence is T2-weighted (long TR and long TE), but the TI is selected to null the signal from CSF.
- The T1 and T2 times of pathologic fluid differs from the signal of CSF.
- For this reason, a diseased tissue exhibits a high signal (hyperintense) and CSF exhibits no signal.
- FLAIR sequences are useful for demonstrating strokes, infections, and white matter disease (Figure 6-10).

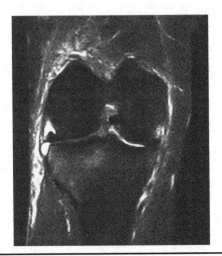

Figure 6-9 A STIR sequence that nulls fat.

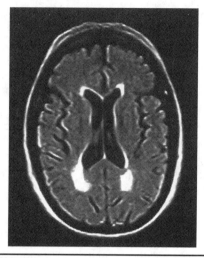

Figure 6-10 A fluid attenuated inversion recovery (FLAIR) sequence, which nulls the cerebrospinal fluid.

- An additional application of inversion sequences is to provide heavy T1 weighting.
- A relatively short TR (1800 to 2000 msec at 1.5 Tesla) is used along with a short TE (≤ 20 msec). The TI is selected once again to null the signal from cerebrospinal fluid (CSF) (≅750 msec at 1.5 Tesla).
- These sequences are useful in pediatric brain examinations. Because white matter is not fully myelinated until 5 years of age, it is difficult to obtain images with good gray-white contrast, particularly with a conventional spin echo sequence. Inversion sequences can provide excellent T1 weighting (Figure 6-11).

In summary, IR sequences provide an excellent tool for optimizing contrast. In the musculoskeletal system, STIR sequences suppress the normal marrow accentuating pathologic fluid. Although STIR sequences suppress or null the signal from fat, it is not specific to fat, and therefore it should not be used in conjunction with gadolinium. Gadolinium shortens the T1 time of hydrogen in water nearly to the T1 time of fat. STIR sequences can suppress the signal from gadolinium thus sup-

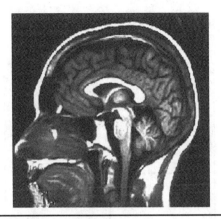

Figure 6-11 A T1-weighted inversion recovery sequence, which may be referred to as T1 FLAIR.

pressing "enhancing" lesions. In brain examinations, FLAIR sequences improve visualization of pathology at CSF interfaces. Inversion sequences can also be used to provide heavily T1-weighted images of the brain. Whatever type of inversion sequence selected, it is important to remember that because TI times are field-strength dependent, the TI required to null a particular tissue is also field-strength dependent. As field strength decreases, the appropriate TI decreases.

IMAGE FORMATION

During the MR acquisition, data is collected by sampling the echo. The data collected during the sampling of the echo (also known as *readout*) is digitized and mapped in relation to the spatial encoding gradients (phase and frequency). This mathematical map is referred to as *k-space*. One direction in k-space represents phase information and the other direction represents frequency information (Figure 6-12).

Physicists often use the letter *k* when referring to frequency. The number of data points in k-space is determined by the number of phase and frequency encodings selected by the operator. The more data points collected during the acquisition, the greater the detail in the resultant image and, in some

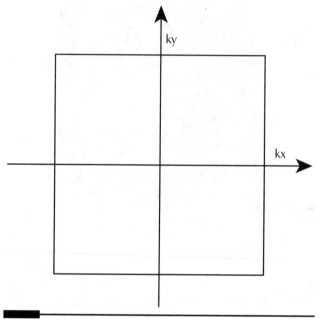

Figure 6-12 K-space. One direction in k-space represents phase information, whereas the other represents frequency.

cases, the longer the scan time. When all the data points have been collected, the MR raw data (k-space data) is sent to the computer, and the image is reconstructed by a mathematical process known as *Fourier transform*. It is important to remember that k-space does not represent the MR image, but rather the data signal information as it relates to the gradient magnetic fields applied during the acquisition process.

An MR image can be considered as having three basic characteristics: contrast, signal-to-noise, and spatial resolution. The contrast is determined by the pulse sequence type and its associated parameters (e.g., TR, TE, TI, flip angle), as well as the tissue's proton density and T1 and T2 (T2*) relaxation times. In this section, we will discuss how the other two characteristics (signal-to-noise and spatial resolution) are dictated.

DATA ACQUISITION

Three main functions are performed during data acquisition: slice selection, phase encoding, and frequency encoding (readout). As mentioned, there are three gradient coils inherent in our system. The purpose of the gradient coils is to produce a magnetic field that varies in intensity in a given direction.

Physical Notation

- The gradient coil oriented to vary the magnetic field in the head-to-foot direction (regardless of the magnetic field orientation) is known as the z gradient.
- The gradient coil oriented to vary the magnetic field in the right-to-left direction is known as the x gradient.
- The gradient coil oriented to vary the magnetic field in the anterior-to-posterior direction is known as the y gradient.

As mentioned, three primary functions are required for MR data collection: slice selection, phase encoding, and frequency encoding. The three gradient coils are capable of performing any of the required functions depending on the choices made by the operator. Generally, when referring to the gradients by function rather than direction or orientation, the logical notation is used.

Logical Notation

- The gradient used to perform slice selection is referred to as the z gradient.
- The gradient used to perform phase encoding is referred to as the y gradient.
- The gradient used to perform frequency encoding is referred to as the x gradient.

A good way to remember the logical notation is to place them in a logical order or alphabetically (x, y, and z). The functions can then be placed in alphabetical order with the corresponding gradient (frequency, phase, and slice).

- When referring to a physical gradient or gradient magnetic field direction, the physical notation is used (Table 6-1).

TABLE 6-1	Physical and Logical Notations Summary	
PHYSICAL NOTATION	LOGICAL NOTATION	GRADIENT
Head/foot	Slice selection	z
Right/left	Phase encoding	y
Anterior/posterior	Frequency encoding	x

- When referring to a particular function of the gradients, the logical notation is used (see Table 6-1).

A simplified pulse sequence diagram (PSD) of a gradient echo sequence demonstrates the application of the gradients in relation to each other over time, labeled as to their function (Figure 6-13). When referring to the function of the gradients, it is important to remember that the logical notation is used.

Slice Selection

- The first gradient to be applied is the slice selection gradient (z).
- The slice selection gradient is "on" during the application of the radio frequency (RF) pulse. In a spin echo sequence, the slice selection gradient is applied during both the 90-degree RF pulse and the 180-degree RF pulse.
- The slice thickness is determined by the amplitude (slope) of the z gradient.
- If a thinner slice is desired, higher amplitude is required. A thicker slice uses lower amplitude.
- The bandwidth of the RF pulse may also be varied to control the slice thickness.
- The slice location is determined by the transmit frequency of the RF pulse (Figure 6-14).

Frequency Encoding

We will skip over the phase encoding gradient at this point and first examine the frequency encoding portion of the data acquisition. To sample the echo, the computer must digitally sample the signal over time. During this sampling, the data points are collected and plotted in k-space.

- If a 256-frequency encoding is selected, the system will sample the echo 256 times in the presence of the frequency encoding gradient.

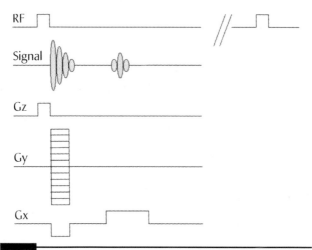

Figure 6-13 A pulse sequence diagram shows the timing of the three major gradients: Gz = slice selection; Gy = phase encoding; Gx = frequency encoding (readout).

- This process will produce 256 data points or frequency "columns" of data, which are plotted in k-space in the frequency or *x* direction (Figure 6-15).
- After one sampling, the computer has only enough data to reconstruct an image with a spatial resolution of 256 × 1.
- If we desire an image with a spatial resolution of 256 × 256, then we must produce 256 echoes, each distinctively encoded for the other direction (*y* direction) in k-space.

Phase Encoding
- The phase encoding (*y* direction) gradient is applied during the free induction decay (FID).
- The purpose of phase encoding is to encode spatial information into the MR signal representing the "line" in k-space on which the data will be plotted during the readout period.
- If a phase resolution of 256 is desired, then the pulse sequence must be repeated a minimum of 256 times.

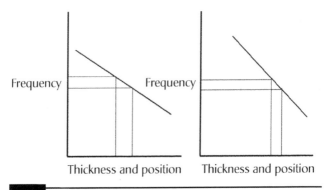

Frequency

Frequency

Thickness and position

Thickness and position

Figure 6-14 The amplitude of the slice selecting gradient (Gz) affects slice thickness. Increasing the amplitude results in a thinner slice excitation.

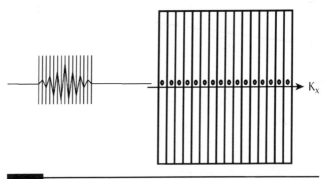

K_x

Figure 6-15 Frequency data are plotted into an K_x direction.

- With each repetition, the phase encoding gradient will be applied with a different amplitude or polarity.
- If 256 phase encodings are prescribed by the operator, then 128 positive steps and 128 negative steps will be applied for a total of 256 steps (Figure 6-16).
- Some vendors refer to the phase encoding steps as *views* or *projections*.
- Spatial resolution may be increased in the phase direction by acquiring a greater number of phase encoding steps.

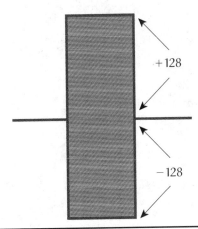

Figure 6-16 If 256-phase encodings are prescribed by the operator, then 128 positive and 128 negative steps, will be applied for a total of 256.

■ Increasing the number of phase encoding steps increases scan time because the pulse sequence must be repeated an equivalent number of times.

In summary, k-space contains the data point acquired during the MR acquisition (Figure 6-17). If 256 phase and 256 frequency encodings are desired, then 256 differently encoded echoes (phase encoding gradient steps) are required. Each echo is sampled 256 times during the readout period (frequency encoding). Although each data point in k-space contains information about the entire image, echoes encoded with high-amplitude phase encoding steps (either positive or negative) are weighted more to spatial resolution or edge detail and resides in the outer edges of k-space. These data points contain little signal information. Echoes encoded with the lower amplitude phase encoding steps are weighted more with signal information and less edge detail. In fact, for 256 lines of k-space data (phase direction), the middle 64 contain over 90% of the image's signal-contrast information.

Figure 6-17 Display of k-space. The higher signal intensity is noted in the central portion, which corresponds to both the low-amplitude phase encodings (phase direction) and the central portion of the echo (frequency direction).

Number of Signal Averages

An additional parameter an MR operator must select is the number of signal averages (NSA). Some MR manufacturers refer to this parameter as the number of excitations (NEX) or acquisitions. NSA can easily be compared with coats of paint on a wall. If all the data points are collected twice and the signals are averaged, then the scan will be performed with two NSA, which will obviously increase the total time of the data acquisition, but does increase the overall signal-to-noise ratio (SNR) of the image.

SCAN TIME

Based on the previous discussion of MR data acquisition, the scan time for a two-dimensional acquisition can be calculated as follows: TR × Ny × NSA, where TR is the pulse repetition time, Ny is the number of phase encodings or views, and NSA is the number of signal averages.

The number of frequency encodings does not affect the scan time because they represent simply the number of digital samples acquired during the brief period in which the echo forms during the readout (a typical sampling time for 256 frequency encodings is 8 msec).

Reducing Scan Time

From the beginning of routine clinical use of MRI, scientists have been working to develop ways to reduce scan time. Faster scan times are not only helpful from the standpoint of patient comfort, but also they allow for acquiring data without the deleterious effects of physiologic motion. Many schemes are used to reduce scan times. For the purpose of this text, we will limit the descriptions to the more common techniques.

Partial Fourier

- Because of the way the data in k-space are encoded, the "upper half" is a mirror image of the "lower half."
- The right and left "halves" are also mirror images.
- Partial Fourier is a technique whereby the top or bottom half of k-space is interpolated based on the values of the data in the other half.
- The top half of k-space is a product of the positive amplitude phase encoding steps. The bottom half is a product of the negative amplitudes (Figure 6-18).
- For example, if we assign an arbitrary phase value of +360 to data obtained following the application of the +128th phase encoding step, then we can expect a value of −360 following the application of the −128th phase encoding step.
- If the +32nd phase encoding step produced data with a phase value of +90, then the −32nd phase encoding step will produce data with a phase value of −90.
- Half Fourier takes advantage of the mathematical symmetry of k-space by acquiring slightly more than one half (either the upper or lower) and then interpolating the data for the other half, similar to the previous example.

Zero Fill

- The centralmost lines of k-space, acquired with the low-amplitude phase encoding steps, contain most of the images' signal and therefore contrast information.

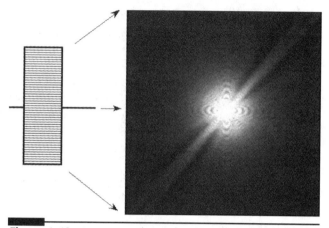

Figure 6-18 The amplitude of the phase encoding gradient relates to date "position" in k-space.

- The outermost lines contain higher spatial or edge detail. Zero fill is a technique that reduces the number of phase encoded steps and therefore reduces the number of lines filled during an acquisition.
- For example, rather than filling all 256 lines (i.e., repeating the pulse sequence 256 times), only the middle 160 lines may be filled.
- The remaining lines, out to 256, are filled with zeros.
- In this example, because only the central 160 lines of k-space are acquired, an image with a resolution of 256 frequency and 160 phase can be reconstructed.
- Some manufacturers may have the operator select a matrix of 256 × 256 and then select a percentage of the matrix to be filled (e.g., 80%). In this case, only the middle 80% of k-space will be filled, and the remaining portion is filled with zeros.
- Because the outermost lines (high-amplitude phase steps) are not acquired, the scan time is reduced at the expense of spatial resolution (Figure 6-19).

Rectangular (Fractional Phase) Field-of-View

Similar to zero fill, rectangular fill results in a reduced scan time but not at the expense of spatial resolution.

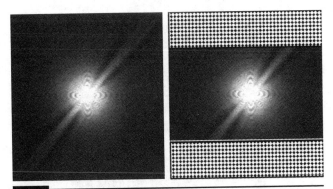

Figure 6-19 **The zero technique.** Scan time is reduced by not filling the higher amplitude (frequency) phase views. Zeros are substituted for the magnetic resonance data. Scan time is reduced at the expense of spatial resolution.

- With rectangular field-of-view (FOV), the number of phase encoding steps is reduced, which reduces scan time.
- Spatial resolution is maintained by reducing the FOV in the phase direction by an equivalent amount.
- Spatial resolution is determined by the voxel volume, which will be discussed in detail later. The pixel size determines the in-plane resolution, determined by dividing the FOV by the number of pixels in the matrix.
- Because the FOV in the phase direction is reduced by an amount equivalent to the reduction in phase encoding steps, the pixel size and therefore spatial resolution remain unchanged.
- The primary penalty for using a rectangular FOV technique is a reduction in signal-to-noise resulting from a reduction in the number of data points sampled.
- Rectangular FOV techniques are useful when the anatomy in the phase direction is smaller than the FOV in that direction.
- As an example, rectangular FOV may be used in an axial T2-weighted acquisition of the brain (Figure 6-20). The phase FOV and the number of phase encoding steps is reduced by a factor of 0.75, resulting in a reduction of scan time without a loss of spatial resolution.

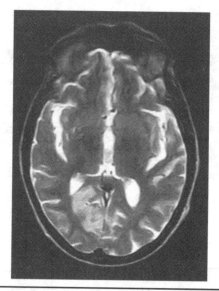

Figure 6-20 The axial sequence of the brain was acquired using a rectangular field of view (FOV). The frequency direction is anterior to posterior, and the phase direction is right to left. The FOV in the frequency direction is 24 and 18 in the phase direction. Since the phase encoding steps were reduced by the same factor (0.75), the scan time was also reduced by a factor of 0.75.

Fast Spin Echo

As previously discussed, the basic principles of data acquisition dictate that if an image with a spatial resolution of 256 frequency and 256 phase is desired, the pulse sequence must be repeated a minimum of 256 times (assuming a full Fourier acquisition). In this acquisition, one echo is produced and sampled during each repetition of the pulse sequence. In other words, one line of k-space is filled during each TR period. Fast spin echo techniques (also known as RARE and turbo spin echo) fill multiple lines of k-space within a single repetition of the pulse sequence. The more lines of k-space filled in a single repetition, the shorter the overall scan time will be.

An analogy may be the writing of a book. If an author decides to write a book with 256 chapters, and each day, he or she writes 1 chapter, then it will take 256 days to complete the book. If three additional authors assist such that four authors were writing the book, then each day, 4 chapters will be written. In this case, it will require only 64 days to complete the book (256 ÷ 4). If eight authors were contributing to the book, then it will take only 32 days to complete the book, since eight chapters will be written each day.

■ In a fast spin echo (FSE) sequence, multiple echoes will be produced within a single repetition of the pulse sequence.

■ The number of echoes produced in a single repetition is an operator-selectable parameter known as the echo train length (ETL) or turbo factor.

■ To "place" each echo in a different line of k-space, a different amplitude of the phase encoding gradient is applied before each echo.

■ Echoes generated following high-amplitude phase encoding gradients are encoded for the outer lines of k-space.

■ Echoes generated following low-amplitude phase encoding gradients are encoded for the inner or central lines of k-space.

■ Because the data points in the central portion of k-space are weighted more toward signal information, they will have a stronger influence on the image contrast.

■ The *effective TE* or *target TE* is the echo that is encoded for the centralmost portion of k-space.

■ The scan time for an FSE sequence is determined using the following formula:

$$\frac{TR \times \text{number of phase encodings} \times NSA}{ETL}$$

A simplified pulse sequence diagram shows an FSE sequence using an 8 ETL (Figure 6-21). In this example, eight lines of k-space will be filled during one TR period. If 256 phase

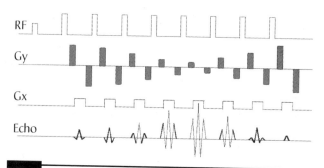

Figure 6-21 A simplified fast spin echo pulse sequence diagram (8 ETL).

encodings were selected (256 phase lines to fill), then the pulse sequence will be repeated a minimum of 32 times, with each echo encoded for 32 lines of k-space. The effective TE will be encoded with the middle 32 phase encoding steps (i.e., ±32).

Controlling Image Quality with Fast Spin Echo

Although FSE has been a tremendous tool for reducing scan times and improving image contrast at both low and high field strengths, it is not without caveats. The primary problem is image blurring. FSE image blurring increases as the effective TE decreases and as the ETL and echo spacing increase.

- Because the rate of T2 decay is exponential, there is greater change in MR signal intensity between echoes early in the train.
- Using a short effective TE places the early echoes in the train in the central portion of k-space.
- The rapid change in signal intensities between echoes mapped to the central portion of k-space results in image blurring.
- As the ETL increases, the effective TE fills less of the central portion of k-space, resulting in echoes of different signal intensities filling the central portion along with the effective TE. As in the previous statements, this factor will result in image blurring (Figure 6-22).

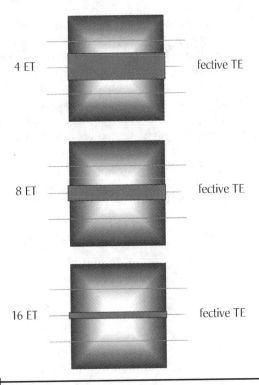

4 ET — fective TE

8 ET — fective TE

16 ET — fective TE

Figure 6-22 The effect of increasing ETL with respect to the number of lines filled by the effective TE. The ETL increases, the effective TE fills less of the center portion of k-space. This results in other echoes filling these "lines." Out of 256 "lines" in k-space, the middle 64 contribute over 90% of an image's contrast and signal information. Increasing the ETL results in the image's contrast being a "composite" of multiple TE times.

The echo spacing is the space or time between each echo. Increasing the echo spacing causes the ETL to extend in time. Because later echoes have a lower signal from T2 decay and as the signal differences between echoes increases, the result is an increase in image blurring. Some manufacturers may provide the operator direct control over the echo spacing while others may allow the operator to control the echo spacing indirectly. In this case, the receive bandwidth is a good way to control the echo spacing. Receive bandwidth will be discussed in more detail later. For the moment, however, increasing the receive bandwidth will reduce the echo spacing thus reducing image blurring. Reducing the receive bandwidth will increase the echo spacing thus increasing image blurring.

In summary, the following steps can be taken to minimize or reduce image blurring that can occur with fast spin echo sequences:

- Increase the effective TE.
- Reduce the ETL.
- Reduce the echo spacing (increase the receive bandwidth).

CHAPTER 7

Magnetic Resonance Image Quality

Chapter at a glance

As previously stated, a magnetic resonance (MR) image can be considered as having three characteristics: contrast, signal-to-noise, and spatial resolution. Having discussed image contrast, we will now examine signal-to-noise and spatial resolution. The difficulty in optimizing MR image quality is that these two characteristics often compete with each other. In most instances, when spatial resolution is increased, signal-to-noise is reduced. Increasing signal-to-noise, depending on the method chosen by the operator, can result in a reduction in spatial resolution.

SPATIAL RESOLUTION

- Spatial resolution is the ability to distinguish one structure from another.

- Voxel volume is a determining factor in spatial resolution.
- The voxel is a three-dimensional object, the size of which is determined by the field-of-view (FOV), acquisition matrix (phase and frequency), and slice thickness.
- The term *pixel* is often applied to the "face" of the voxel, which is determined by the FOV and the acquisition matrix.
- Pixel size is synonymous with the term *in-plane* resolution.
- To determine the pixel size, (1) divide the FOV (in units of mm) by the frequency matrix, (2) divide the FOV (in units of mm) by the phase matrix, and (3) multiply the answers from steps 1 and 2. The answer will be in units of square millimeters (mm²).
- To determine the voxel volume, (1) divide the FOV (in units of mm) by the frequency matrix, (2) divide the FOV (in units of mm) by the phase matrix, and (3) multiply the answer from steps 1 by the answer from 2 and then multiply this product by the slice thickness. The answer will be in units of cubic millimeters (mm³) (Figure 7-1).
- The FOV controls the voxel volume (as demonstrated in the previous calculation), but it is important to remember that the FOV controls the voxel volume in two dimensions.
- If the operator reduces the FOV by 20%, the voxel volume decreases by 40%.

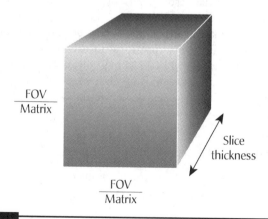

Figure 7-1 Parameters used in calculating the voxel volume.

- Using a larger FOV and then magnifying the image for photographic purposes (making the image larger on the film) does not increase spatial resolution.
- The only way to increase spatial resolution is to reduce the voxel volume or pixel size.
- Magnification can make the image appear blurry because it magnifies the pixel.

Signal-to-Noise

The term signal-to-noise refers to a ratio of MR signal-to-noise. Noise is random and originates from multiple sources, including the environment, the patient, and the system's electronics. Signal comes only from the patient, or more specifically, the tissue in the voxel. To increase the signal-to-noise ratio (SNR), the technologist must increase the signal or reduce the noise. All operator-selectable acquisition parameters affect the SNR. Surface coils are also powerful tools for increasing the SNR. The following text explores the effect of various parameters on the SNR. For the purposes of this discussion, an assumption is made that all other parameters will remain unchanged. For example, when describing the effect of increasing the repetition time (TR), the assumption will be made that all other parameters will be unchanged.

Timing Parameters

- Increasing the TR increases the amount of longitudinal magnetization allowed to recover between excitation periods (TR) and will therefore result in an increase in the SNR.
- Reducing the TR will increase the saturation of tissues and will therefore result in a reduction in the SNR.
- Increasing the time to the echo (TE) increases the amount of transverse magnetization decay between the excitation pulse and the sampling of the echo. The result is a reduction in the SNR.
- Reducing the TE reduces the amount of transverse magnetization decay between the excitation pulse and the sampling of the echo. Again, the result is an increase in the SNR.

- Increasing or reducing the inversion time (TI) is not as straightforward. However, if the decision is made, for example, to null the signal from fat, and the area being imaged contains a large amount of fat, then the resultant image will be a rather low SNR because the major tissue providing the signal (in this example, fat) is nulled.

Flip Angle

Adjusting the flip angle of a gradient echo sequence can either increase or decrease the SNR of an image, depending on other parameters. With extremely low flip angles (e.g., 5 degrees), the amount of transverse magnetization is rather small as is the resultant SNR. In this example, increasing the flip angle from that point will increase the SNR. There will be a point, however, when the signal will reach its maximum and will then begin to decrease as the flip angle continues to be increased. The flip angle that produces the maximal signal for a given tissue at a given TR is known as the *Ernst angle*.

- If the flip angle is below the Ernst angle, then increasing the flip angle will result in an increase in the SNR and vice versa.
- If the flip angle is greater than the Ernst angle, then increasing the flip angle will result in a reduction in the SNR and vice versa.
- The Ernst angle will be specific for various tissues and is based on the TR and the T1 time of the tissue.

Voxel Volume

As previously discussed, voxel volume controls the spatial resolution. Voxel volume also directly affects the SNR. In fact, the SNR is directly proportional to the voxel volume.

- Increasing the slice thickness will increase the SNR.
- Reducing the slice thickness will reduce the SNR.
- For example, if the slice thickness is increased from 3 to 6 mm, then the voxel volume will double, thus the SNR will increase by a factor of two (doubled).
- Increasing the number of phase or frequency encodings reduces voxel volume and reduces the SNR.
- Reducing the number of phase or frequency encodings increases voxel volume and increases the SNR.

- Increasing the FOV increases voxel volume and increases the SNR.
- Reducing the FOV reduces voxel volume and reduces the SNR.
- The FOV has the greatest effect on voxel volume because it affects the voxel size in two dimensions.
- For example, if the FOV is increased by only 20%, then the voxel volume will be increased by 40% (20% in each direction). As a result, the SNR will increase by a factor of 40%.

Sampling Parameters

The term *sampling parameters* refers to parameters that control the amount of time spent sampling the MR signal. One may also say that the sampling parameters control the number of samples taken during the MR data acquisition. These parameters include number of signal averages (NSA), phase encodings, frequency encodings, and receiver bandwidth. Generally, when more time is spent collecting signal, noise increases. However, noise is random such that, if the number of signal averages is doubled, the SNR does not double because of the random increase of noise.

Number of Signal Averages

- The NSA is somewhat analogous to coats of paint.
- For example, if an MR scan is acquired with two NSA, each line of k-space is filled twice and the signals are averaged.
- Again, because noise increases randomly, the SNR is proportional to the $\sqrt{NSA}$
- In this example, the total scan time is twice that of a scan acquired with one NSA.
- The SNR, however, will not double, but rather, increase by $\sqrt{2}$.

As the relationship between SNR and NSA indicates, to double the SNR (i.e., to increase the SNR by a factor of two), the NSA will have to be increased by a factor of four ($\sqrt{4} = 2$). As mentioned, since increasing the NSA by a factor of four results in a four-fold increase in sampling time, the total scan time increases by a factor of four. Generally, attempting to increase the SNR by increasing the NSA is inefficient from the perspective of scan time (Figure 7-2).

$$\text{Original NSA} = 2$$
$$\text{New NSA} = 4$$

$$\text{New NSA} = \sqrt{\dfrac{\text{New NSA}}{\text{Original NSA}}}$$

$$\text{New NSA} = \sqrt{\dfrac{4}{2}} = \sqrt{2} = 1.41$$

Figure 7-2 Formula calculates the effects of changing the NSA on the SNR.

Number of Phase Encoding and Frequency Encoding Steps

- Increasing the number of phase or frequency encoding steps also increases the number of samples taken during an acquisition.
- The SNR is proportional to $\sqrt{\text{total sampling time}}$. Therefore increasing the number of samples by this method increases the SNR.
- An increase in the number of phase or frequency samples also reduces the voxel volume.
- The SNR is directly proportional to voxel volume. Therefore the net effect on the SNR when the phase and/or frequency samples is increased is a reduction in the SNR.
- In other words, the effect from the reduction in voxel volume is greater than the effect from the increase in sampling time.

Receiver Bandwidth

The receiver bandwidth represents the range of frequencies sampled during the application of the frequency encoding (readout) gradient. Receiver bandwidth is determined by the number of frequency samples to be taken (frequency matrix) and the time required to take these samples. For example, if 256 frequency samples are collected (i.e., a 256-frequency matrix) and the readout or sampling period is 8 milliseconds, then the receiver bandwidth will be 16 kHz (or an absolute bandwidth of 32 kHz). The relationship between the number of samples, the sampling time, and the receiver bandwidth is illustrated in Figure 7-3.

$$\text{Receiver bandwidth} = \frac{\text{Frequency matrix (sample)}}{\text{Readout (sampling) time}}$$

$$32 \text{ kHz} = \frac{256}{8}$$

Figure 7-3 The relationship among the number of samples, the sampling time, and the receiver bandwidth.

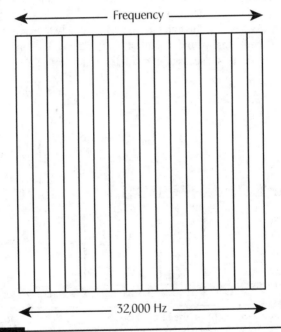

← Frequency →

← 32,000 Hz →

Figure 7-4 The receiver bandwidth is mapped across the field of view in the frequency direction.

■ At a field strength of 1.5 Tesla, the center frequency is 42.6 MHz/T × 1.5 T or 63.9 MHz.

■ With a receiver bandwidth of 32kHz, the frequencies sampled will be 63.9 MHz ±16 kHz.

■ The frequencies sampled are "mapped" across the FOV, as illustrated in Figure 7-4.

Because noise is random and occurs at the upper and lower ranges of the bandwidth, if the receiver bandwidth is reduced, then the noise will be reduced, resulting in a greater SNR.

- Reducing the receiver bandwidth reduces the noise, thereby increasing the SNR (Figure 7-5).
- The reduction in bandwidth, however, has its consequences.
- To satisfy the Nyquist theorem, the sampling time must be increased as the bandwidth decreases.
- For example, if the receiver bandwidth is changed from 32 kHz to 16 kHz (-8 kHz), as shown in the following calculation, then the sampling (readout) time ($+8$ kHz) increases from 8 to 16 msec.
- As a result, the minimum TE attainable will increase.
- Additionally, the chemical shift artifact will increase (which is discussed in detail later) (Figure 7-6).

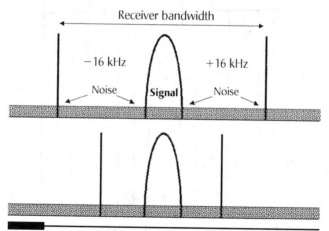

Figure 7-5 Reducing the receiver bandwidth reduces the amount of noise relative to the magnetic resonance signal.

$$32 \text{ kHz} = \frac{256}{8 \text{ msec}} \qquad 16 \text{ kHz} = \frac{256}{16 \text{ msec}}$$

Figure 7-6 The effect of receiver bandwidth on sampling time.

- Because a chemical shift artifact is significantly less at lower field strengths, reducing the receiver bandwidth to improve the SNR is used more often on lower field strength systems (0.5 Tesla or less).

Surface Coils

As mentioned, the primary purpose of local (surface) coils is to improve the SNR. A smaller coil will produce a higher SNR, although less tissue is imaged (with the exception of a phased-array configuration). The SNR can be optimized with surface coils by selecting a coil that is "sized" for the anatomy being imaged.

Three-Dimensional Acquisitions

Two primary techniques are used for acquiring image data: two-dimensional Fourier transform (2-DFT) and three-dimensional Fourier transform (3-DFT). A 2-D acquisition excites a slice of tissue selectively, and a 3-D acquisition excites a slab of tissue. Because a thick slab would provide inadequate spatial resolution, the slab is partitioned into slices by a phase encoding gradient applied in the slice (z) direction. The number of slice encoding steps applied determines the number of partitions (slices). Increasing the number of partitions through a given slab decreases the thickness of the resultant slice. For example, if a 120-mm slab were acquired with 60 phase encodings in the slice (z) direction, then the result will be 60 images, each having a slice thickness of 2 mm. If the number of slice encodings were increased to 120, then the result will be 120 images, each with a slice thickness of 1 mm (Figure 7-7).

- Scan time for a 3-D acquisition is given by TR $\times$ Ny $\times$ NSA $\times$ the number of slices.
- For this reason, the 120-partition data set previously described will have twice the acquisition time of the 60-partition data set.
- However, because SNR is proportional to the $\sqrt{\text{total sampling time}}$, the 120-partition data set will have $\sqrt{2}$ greater SNR.

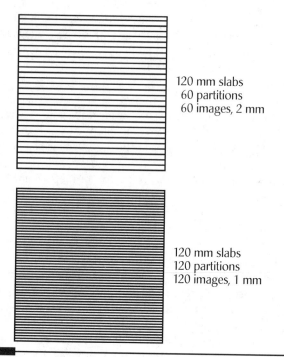

120 mm slabs
60 partitions
60 images, 2 mm

120 mm slabs
120 partitions
120 images, 1 mm

Figure 7-7 Increasing the number of slice encoding.

This property demonstrates the power of a 3-D acquisition; the more slice encodings for a given slab size, the thinner the resultant slices and the higher the SNR.

Isotropic Voxels

If a 3-D data set is acquired with isotropic voxels, the data set may be reformatted to produce images in any plane.

- An isotropic voxel is equal in all dimensions (i.e., a cube).
- To prescribe an isotropic data set, the operator should first select a square matrix (256 frequency and 256 phase).

> Matrix of 256 = 256, field of view = 280 mm
> 280 ÷ 256 = 1.1
>
> 1.1 mm should be selected as the slice thickness
> (partition thickness)

Figure 7-8 Isotropic voxel calculation example.

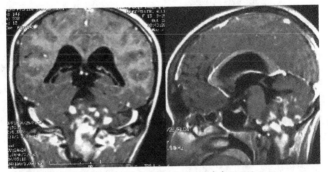

Figure 7-9 Reformatted images of an axial data set.

- The next step is to divide the FOV, in millimeter units, by the matrix.
- The result should be selected as the slice thickness (Figure 7-8).

As a practical matter, most workstations interpolate 3-D data sets such that voxels need not be exactly isotropic. Generally, the FOV is divided by the phase encoding matrix. The result of this calculation is then chosen for the slice thickness. Even then, the operator may adjust the slice thickness slightly (typically ±0.2 mm).

The coronal and sagittal images in Figure 7-9 are reformatted images of an axial data set, which were acquired at 0.2 T with a scan time of 5.5 minutes.

The parameters, including their effect on SNR, spatial resolution, and scan time, are summarized in Table 7-1.

TABLE 7-1 Parameter Effects

PARAMETER	SNR	SPATIAL RESOLUTION	SCAN TIME
Increase TR	Increase	N/A	Increase
Reduce TR	Reduce	N/A	Reduce
Increase TE	Reduce	N/A	N/A
Reduce TE	Increase	N/A	N/A
Increase receiver bandwidth	Reduce	N/A	N/A
Reduce receiver bandwidth	Increase	N/A	N/A
Increase FOV	Increase	Reduce	N/A
Reduce FOV	Reduce	Increase	N/A
Increase slice thickness	Increase	Reduce	N/A
Reduce slice thickness	Reduce	Increase	N/A
Increase frequency matrix	Reduce	Increase	N/A
Reduce frequency matrix	Increase	Reduce	N/A
Increase NSA	Increase	N/A	Increase
Reduce NSA	Reduce	N/A	Reduce
Increase number of 3-D partitions (maintain slab size)	Increase	Increase	Increase
Reduce number of 3-D partitions (maintain slab size)	Reduce	Reduce	Reduce

FOV, Field of view; *NSA,* number signal averages; *SNR, TE,* echo time; *TR,* repetition time.

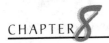
Artifacts

Chapter at a glance

An artifact may be described as anything appearing on a magnetic resonance (MR) image that does not exist in the area being imaged. Technologists must learn to recognize artifacts and know what can be done to reduce or eliminate them. MR artifacts can be subdivided into several categories. The physical principles of MR contribute to the presence of artifacts. Sampling artifacts are a result of techniques used to sample the MR signal. Equipment artifacts are a result of malfunctioning equipment or its failure.

CHEMICAL SHIFT

■ As mentioned, hydrogen in fat and hydrogen in water precess at different frequencies.

- This difference in resonant frequency is referred to as chemical shift.

- Chemical shift is field-strength dependent and increases with field strength.

- Additionally, as we sample the echo, the frequencies are "mapped" across the field-of-view (FOV) in the frequency direction.

- Receive bandwidth determines the Hertz/pixel value.

- Because fat and water differ in frequency, a pixel shift occurs at fat and water interfaces.

- At 1.5 Tesla, for example, if 256 frequency encodings are selected, and if the receive bandwidth is 32 kHz, then each pixel will be 125 Hz apart. Because fat and water are separated by 224 Hz at 1.5 Tesla, fat and water will be shifted 1.8 pixels.

- Using the previous example, if the receive bandwidth were reduced to 16 kHz, the Hertz/pixel value will be 62.5 Hz/pixel. Because the chemical shift at 1.5 Tesla is 224 Hz, the pixel shift in this case will be 3.6 pixels.

- The chemical shift artifact appears as a black or white band at fat and water interfaces and occurs in the frequency direction.

- Reducing the receiver bandwidth causes the chemical shift artifact to increase (greater pixel shift).

- Increasing the receiver bandwidth causes the chemical shift artifact to decrease (less pixel shift).

- A chemical shift artifact is an example of an artifact that cannot be eliminated but can be reduced.

- As the field strength decreases, the chemical shift artifact becomes less apparent.

CHEMICAL SHIFT OF THE SECOND KIND

- Gradient echo sequences do not have the 180-degree radio-frequency (RF) pulse before the echo as in spin echo sequences.

- As such, gradient recalled echo (GRE) sequences do not correct for slight inhomogeneities and chemical shifts.

- At an echo time (TE) of zero (i.e., immediately following the creation of transverse magnetization) fat and water spins are in phase.

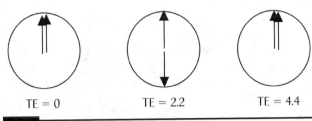

Figure 8-1 At 1.5 Tesla, fat and water spins cycle in and out of phase every 2.2 millisecond.

■ As time passes, water spins will gain phase relative to the fat spins because of their slightly higher precessional frequency.

■ Within a few milliseconds, the water spins will "catch up" to the fat spins, and once again, fat and water will be in phase.

■ The timing of this cycling of the spins is field-strength dependent (as chemical shift is field-strength dependent).

■ At 1.5 Tesla, fat and water spins cycle in and out of phase every 2.2 msec (Figure 8-1).

■ When a voxel containing both fat and water is imaged at a TE when fat and water are 180 degrees out of phase, the vectors will cancel and produce a signal void in that voxel.

■ A GRE sequence acquired with fat and water out of phase will exhibit a dark line at fat and water interfaces.

■ To correct for this result (i.e., to eliminate the dark line), the operator should select a TE with fat and water in phase.

■ To calculate the increment of phase cycling, the following formula can be used.

$$\frac{1}{\text{Field strength}} \times 3.355$$

Example for 1.5 T

$$\frac{1}{1.5} \times 3.355 = 2.2$$

TE = 0 in phase
TE = 2.2 out of phase
TE = 4.4 in phase

Table 8-1 offers in-phase and out-of-phase TE times for various field strengths.

This particular phenomenon is not observed with spin echo techniques because the 180-degree refocusing pulse corrects for this manifestation of chemical shift.

Magnetic Susceptibility

■ Magnetic susceptibility refers to the property of a substance to become magnetized.

■ Metal objects in the body are magnetized to a greater extent compared with the surrounding tissues.

■ The effect on the spins in the area of the metal object is such that they experience a different magnetic field because of the presence of the metal.

■ As a result, the spins in close proximity to the metal precess at a frequency vastly different from the spins farther away from the metal.

■ The spins in the area of the metal are therefore not affected by the excitation pulse because of their frequency.

■ The result is a signal void in the area of the metal.

■ If a gradient echo sequence is used for the acquisition, this type of area will exhibit a greater loss of signal compared with a spin echo acquisition of the same area.

■ The 180-degree radio frequency (RF) pulse used in a spin echo sequence will correct for some of the inhomogeneities created by the metal. Although a signal void can still be observed in the immediate area of the metal, it will be smaller than the void produced with a gradient echo sequence.

Table 8-1 In- and Out-of-Phase TE Times

FIELD STRENGTH	IN-PHASE TE	OUT-OF-PHASE TE	IN-PHASE TE
0.2 T	0	17.0	34.0
0.3 T	0	11.0	22.0
1.0 T	0	3.3	6.6
1.5 T	0	2.2	4.4

T, Tesla; TE, echo time.

- To further reduce the size of the signal void, fast spin echo (FSE) sequences can be used. The multiple 180-degree pulses used in FSE sequences greatly reduce magnetic susceptibility effects reducing the overall size of the signal void.

- As a clinical matter, it has long been known that GRE sequences are far superior to spin echo sequences (and to a greater extent, FSE sequences) for sensitivity to hemorrhage, particularly in the brain.

- When a hemorrhage breaks down over time, hemosiderin remains, which is an intracellular storage form of iron thus producing a small local inhomogeneity.

- The 180-degree pulse corrects for this local inhomogeneity to the extent that it may not be visible with spin echo-based sequences.

- The presence of metal or hemorrhage is not the only source for signal loss caused by susceptibility effects.

- In the body, tissues vary in their magnetic susceptibility.

- For example, air is hardly magnetized while tissue such as brain have a relatively high magnetization.

- When two tissues with different magnetic susceptibilities, such as air and brain matter interface, a small local gradient magnetic field is created.

- Again, spin echo-based sequences largely correct for this inhomogeneity, whereas gradient echo-based sequences do not.

- Regardless of whether spin echo or GRE sequences are used, magnetic susceptibility artifacts can be affected by several parameters.

- Magnetic susceptibility is proportional to field strength, voxel volume, and TE.

- As field strength decreases, magnetic susceptibility decreases.

- As voxel volume decreases, magnetic susceptibility decreases.

- As TE is reduced, magnetic susceptibility is decreased.

- For these reasons, signal loss from magnetic susceptibility effects is less of a problem with low field strength systems.
- 3-D GRE sequences that use small voxels and short TE times will also have fewer artifacts from magnetic susceptibility as compared with 2-D sequences that use larger voxels (and possibly longer TE times).

Motion and Flow

Magnetic resonance imaging (MRI) uses gradient magnetic fields to encode the signals to derive spatial information. Any movement of spins can cause artifacts and loss of signal. The cause of motion artifacts and imaging options that may be used to reduce or eliminate them will be briefly described.

- Motion of tissues during the acquisition process is observed as a smearing or *ghosting* along the phase encoding direction.
- This effect is primarily a result of movement of spins following the application of the phase encoding gradient and the inherent time delay to the sampling or readout of the signal.
- Motion is generally not observed in the frequency encoding direction because of the usually short duration of the readout gradient and the fact that frequency encoding is performed during this readout period.
- Various techniques can be used to reduce or eliminate ghosting, depending on the type of motion or its origin.
- Motion can be subdivided into two main types: periodic and aperiodic.
- Periodic motion is characterized by motion that occurs at somewhat regular intervals.
- Examples of periodic motion include respiration, cardiac motion, blood flow, and CSF pulsation.
- Aperiodic motion is characterized by motion that occurs at irregular or random intervals.
- Examples of aperiodic motion include swallowing, peristalsis, and general body motion.
- Compensating for periodic motion is easier because the movement can be somewhat predictable.

SPATIAL PRESATURATION

In a spin echo sequence, flowing blood generally produces a signal void, because both the 90-degree and the 180-degree RF pulses are slice-selective. Flowing blood that receives a 90-degree RF pulse is not in the slice to receive the 180-degree pulse and thus produces no MR signal. In a multislice sequence, however, blood moves through multiple slice locations and receives multiple RF pulses. As a result, phase mismapping occurs. To reduce this artifact and produce images demonstrating signal void in vessels with flowing blood, additional RF pulses can be applied to the blood as it enters the imaging volume.

The term saturation implies reduction in MR signal. Spins are saturated when they are given insufficient time to regain longitudinal magnetization between excitation pulses. Saturated spins will produce little or no MR signal. In the case of flowing blood, a 90-degree RF pulse is applied outside the imaging volume (range of slices). When the blood flows into the imaging volume, it has minimal or no longitudinal magnetization as a result of the 90-degree pulse. When the 90-degree pulse is applied in a slice, the blood in that slice has no longitudinal magnetization that can be directed to the transverse plane and thus no MR signal is produced.

- Presaturation pulses are generally applied outside the imaging volume in the direction of blood flow.
- For example, when acquiring axial images of the neck and a hypointense signal in blood vessels is desired, presaturation pulses can be prescribed superior and inferior to the slice group.
- Because it is generally desirable to acquire spin echo sequences such that flowing blood produces no signal in the vessels, presaturation pulses are often prescribed in the direction of blood flow (typically superior and inferior).
- Using presaturation pulses with spin echo pulse sequences provides an excellent technique for demonstrating clot and extremely slow blood flow within vessels.
- Clot and extremely slow flow will appear as hyperintense relative to fast flow from blood receiving both the 90-degree and 180-degree pulse.

Gradient Moment Nulling

Generally, motion during an MR acquisition causes a reduction or loss of MR signal. However, it is often desirable to acquire images with bright signal from flowing blood, which can be accomplished by use of a technique known as gradient moment nulling (GMN). Other names used for this technique include flow compensation, gradient moment reduction (GMR), and motion artifact suppression technique (MAST).

- GMN, specifically first-order GMN, adds extra lobes to the frequency and slice selection gradients before sampling the echo.
- The effect is to regain phase coherence lost by moving spins, which, in turn, will produce vessels with bright signal.
- First-order GMN corrects only for constant velocity (i.e., slow, pulsatile flow) but does not correct for complex motions such as accelerated flow and jerk.
- GMN works best when short TE times are used because it reduces the time between excitation and readout.
- GMN can also be used to reduce flow artifacts caused by CSF pulsations on T2- or T2*-weighted sequences.
- These pulsations may cause ghosting artifacts in the base of the skull on brain examinations and loss of signal in cervical spine examinations.

Compensation for Respiration

- The simplest way to compensate for respiratory motion is to eliminate it.
- Advances in hardware and software technology now make it possible to acquire sequences with such short scan times that they can be acquired during a breath-hold.
- Breath-hold sequences can now be acquired on most systems using either GRE or fast spin echo sequences.
- In some cases, the artifact can be redirected such that the ghosting does not enter the anatomy of interest.
- For example, when imaging the cervical spine, if the phase encoding direction is anterior-to-posterior, any ghosting artifact caused by swallowing motion will be directed through the vertebral bodies and the spinal cord.

- The artifact can be redirected by swapping the direction of the phase encoding gradient to the superior-to-inferior (head-to-foot) direction. Because the artifact is originating from motion in the anterior neck, the artifact will be redirected superior-to-inferior and anterior to the area of interest.
- As an option, spatial presaturation pulses can be prescribed within the imaging FOV to remove unwanted signal.
- If the tissue is saturated, it produces little, if any, signal and thus the ghosting artifacts are reduced.

Respiratory motion artifacts are also reduced by the use of either respiratory compensation or respiratory triggering. Both techniques usually require the use of a type of belt placed around the patient's abdomen or chest to detect the respiratory motion.

- Respiratory compensation, also known as ROPE (respiratory ordered phase encoding), "maps" the respiration cycles of the patient and alters the order of the phase encoding steps.
- Typically, phase encodings are applied linearly (i.e., going from maximal positive to maximal negative).
- Respiratory compensation will perform the low-amplitude phase steps (highest signal weighting, middle of k-space) during the period between breaths. The outer phase encoding steps are acquired during the period of maximal motion.
- The more evenly a patient breathes, the better the artifact suppression will be.
- With respiratory compensation, the repetition time (TR) remains as set by the operator.
- Respiratory triggering does not alter the order of the phase encoding steps but uses the patient's respiration cycle to trigger the scan for each TR (similar to cardiac gating).
- As such, the TR is dependent on the patient's respiratory rate and is not subject to a great deal of control by the operator.
- In either case, the respiratory artifacts are, at best, minimized but not eliminated.
- The use of phased-array coils for abdominal and pelvic imaging will improve the signal-to-noise ratio (SNR), but

the presence of a coil on the anterior abdominal wall will greatly increase the signal from the surface tissues. This coil position can cause the signal from the respiratory "ghosts" to appear more intense.

■ Spectral fat suppression techniques are sometimes used in abdominal imaging to enhance lesion conspicuity on T1- or T2-weighted sequences. A by-product of fat suppression is a reduction in respiratory ghosting artifacts resulting from the reduction of the signal from fat.

CARDIAC COMPENSATION

To produce images of the heart, it is necessary to either scan so quickly as to eliminate cardiac motion or to trigger the acquisition with the cardiac cycle.

■ The patient first has electrocardiogram (ECG) electrodes and leads applied.

■ The cardiac cycle is detected either by hardware built into the MR computer or by an external monitor connected to the MR computer.

■ The excitation pulse for each TR is triggered by the R wave of the cardiac cycle.

■ Each slice is excited at the same point during the cardiac cycle, greatly reducing the effects of cardiac motion.

■ As with respiratory triggering, the TR is controlled by the patients' heart rate or the R-R interval (Figure 8-2).

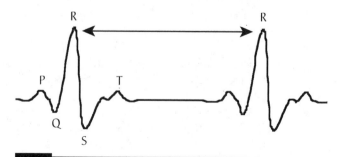

Figure 8-2 To produce images of the heart, it is necessary to either scan so fast to eliminate cardiac motion or to trigger the acquisition with the cardiac cycle.

- The QRS complex represents ventricular contraction (systole). The QRS interval, in electrocardiography, is the interval from the beginning of the Q wave to the termination of the S wave, representing the time for ventricular depolarization.
- The R wave triggers the scan.
- Scanning takes place between the R-R interval, which is now the TR.
- If the patient has a heart rate of 60 beats per minute, the scan will be triggered 60 times per minute or every second. The effective TR will therefore be 1 second or 1000 msec.
- Depending on the MR system, the operator may have to program delay times, which are played out after the R wave.
- In this case, the actual time available for imaging will be equal to the R-R interval minus any delay times.

Cardiac gating may be used to acquire images of the heart or simply to reduce ghosting caused by cardiac motion. Cerebral spinal fluid (CSF) pulsation is associated with cardiac motion. Cardiac gating may also be used to reduce CSF signal loss caused by pulsatile motion during examinations of the spine and brain (Figure 8-3).

APERIODIC MOTION

Respiratory motion and cardiac motion are examples of periodic motion in that they occur at relatively consistent intervals. Aperiodic motion has no such consistency. Examples are bowel peristalsis and general patient motion.

- Bowel peristalsis can often be reduced by using antispasmodic drugs such as glucagon.
- Application of binding straps across the abdomen can also reduce the effects of peristalsis but may be uncomfortable for the patient or increase their anxiety about the procedure.
- Imaging the patient in the prone position is another technique that can be used to reduce the effects of peristalsis.

Patient motion can be the most frustrating problem to address. Advances in MR hardware and software technology have made it possible to acquire data in scan times of 1 minute

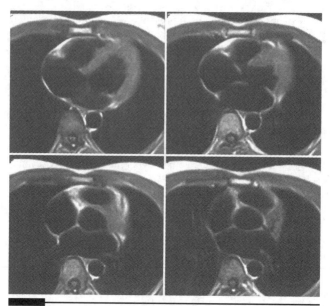

Figure 8-3 Cardiac gating may be used to acquire images of the heart or simply to reduce ghosting caused by cardiac motion.

compared with the 17 minutes it used to take. Nevertheless, if the patient is not comfortable, then movement during the examination is highly likely.

- Therefore the first step in reducing patient motion is to make the patient comfortable.
- The use of tape and restraint straps may appear to be a good idea, and in some cases, may actually be the method of choice. For patients who are able to cooperate, however, they may only serve to increase their level of anxiety about the procedure.
- Sponges can be used to support and restrain the patient without them feeling as though they are "trapped" in the magnet.
- Aperiodic and even periodic motion artifacts can also be reduced by increasing the number of signal averages (NSA).
- Sedation and even general anesthesia can be used to solve patient motion problems. However, these meas-

ures will increase the risk to the patient and require additional patient monitoring procedures and protocols to be in place.

Aliasing

Also known as a *fold-over* or *wrap-around* artifact, aliasing occurs when tissue that is excited by the RF pulse falls outside the FOV. Aliasing is an example of a sampling artifact and occurs in both the phase and frequency directions. Since it is easily and transparently compensated for in the frequency direction on most state-of-the-art systems, we will focus on aliasing in the phase direction.

- During data acquisition, the phase encoding gradient encodes phase shifts from −360 degrees to +360 degrees across the prescribed FOV.
- Excited tissue that falls outside the FOV has a phase shift of greater than −360 degrees and/or +360 degrees and thus has a phase value already "assigned" to a location within the FOV.
- For example, the tissue at one edge of the FOV has a phase value of +360 degrees. A tissue with a phase value of +370 degrees lies just beyond the FOV.
- To the computer, the phase value of +370 degrees reads as the phase value of +10 degrees and as such, both are reconstructed and displayed in the same location.
- Essentially, this effect results in tissue from just outside the right side of the FOV to be folded over and superimposed over tissue inside the left side of the FOV and vice versa (assuming a right-to-left phase encoding direction).
- The first and simplest way to compensate for this artifact is to increase the FOV. Although this will reduce or even remove the aliased signal, it will also reduce the spatial resolution.
- The second technique is known as *oversampling*.
- An oversampling technique will increase the FOV in the phase direction and increase the number of phase encoding steps simultaneously to maintain spatial resolution.
- The image is reconstructed and displayed with the prescribed FOV.

- Although this technique will not reduce the spatial resolution, it will increase scan time.
- To overcome the effect on scan time, the NSA can be decreased, which can be done either manually or automatically, depending on the system software.
- For example, if a sequence is acquired with a 24 FOV, 256 matrix, and 4 NSA, then prescribing an oversampling technique (100%) will increase the FOV to 48 and the phase matrix to 512. If the NSA is reduced to two, the pixel size and the scan time will remain the same. The image is reconstructed with the originally prescribed 24 FOV.

GIBBS AND TRUNCATION ARTIFACT

Although two separate types of artifacts, Gibbs and truncation artifacts are both sampling artifacts that have similar appearances and both can be reduced by increasing the number of phase encoding steps.

- Truncation artifacts occur when tissues are undersampled along the phase encoding direction, and these tissues have different signal amplitudes (i.e., interfaces with high and low signal intensities, such as in a sagittal, T2-weighted sequence through the cervical spine).
- Truncation and Gibbs artifacts appear as striations or lines in the phase direction, corresponding with the high and low signal interface.
- A good example of this artifact can be observed on a sagittal cervical spine sequence with the phase encoding direction anterior-to-posterior. Truncation will appear as a line (or lines) within the spinal cord.
- On a sagittal, T1-weighted cervical spine sequence, the artifact will appear as a low signal-intensity line within the higher signal intensity of the spinal cord. On a sagittal, T2-weighted cervical spine sequence, the artifact will appear as a high signal-intensity line within the lower signal intensity of the spinal cord.
- Increasing the number of phase encoding steps will not remove the artifact; it will only make it less obvious.

RADIO-FREQUENCY ARTIFACTS

■ RF artifacts are also known as *zipper* artifacts.

■ As implied, RF artifacts appear as a bright and dark band running through the image.

■ These artifacts are a result of an extraneous RF signal detected by the receiver coil.

■ Common causes include a leak in the RF shielding.

■ RF leaks may come from scanning with the scan room door opened or not tightly closed.

■ Leaks may also originate from electrical current coming into or originating within the scan room.

■ Equipment such as patient monitoring devices that are not actually MR compatible can be the cause of RF artifacts.

■ Holes or tears in the RF shielding can result in extraneous signals entering the scan room and manifesting themselves as zipper artifacts on images.

■ Whatever the cause, an effort should be made to locate the source of the signals and either correct or remove it.

GRADIENT MALFUNCTIONS

■ Nonlinearity of gradient magnetic fields can result in images with a mild or gross distortion of normal anatomy.

■ The cause is generally a failure of the electronics or software controlling the gradient magnetic fields.

■ Repeated occurrences require that the system be turned over to the service engineer for service or calibration.

IMAGE SHADING

■ Shading is described as an inhomogeneous signal across an image when using a single coil to encompass the anatomy being imaged.

■ Shading is more commonly described as loss of signal in one or more areas toward the edge of the anatomy.

■ Shading usually requires intervention by the service engineer.

Inadequate System Tuning

- Nearly every MR system requires the operator to perform some type of "tuning" before scanning.

- This so-called *prescan* can include tuning the system to the resonant frequency of the patient (sometimes referred to as *center frequency*).

- Prescan tuning can also include determining the proper amount of RF energy necessary to "tip" the net magnetization 90 degrees.

- With some systems, the receiver coil may also have to be adjusted for optimal impedance matching or loading.

- Most current systems perform these prescan tuning procedures automatically.

- However, when the automatic prescan algorithm fails or when manual tuning is not properly performed, images with inadequate quality will likely be produced.

- Symptoms can include images with severe shading, low SNR, or tissue contrasts that appear to be reversed.

- The remedy is to either properly perform the prescan tuning procedures or, in the case of a failure in the automatic prescan algorithm, have the service engineer check the system calibration.

Reconstruction Artifacts

- When the MR data are collected, they are sent to the array processor to undergo the final Fourier transform calculations.

- Because Fourier transform is a mathematical process, errors occurring during the data collection or reconstruction process have a distinctive appearance.

- Generally, reconstruction artifacts appear as geometric patterns superimposed on or across the image.

- Examples of reconstruction artifacts include the so-called *corduroy* and *herringbone* artifacts.

- Extraneous RF signals can also produce artifacts that appear similar to reconstruction artifacts.

- Whatever the cause, repeated occurrences require the attention of the service engineer.

Flow Imaging

Chapter at a glance

FLOW PATTERNS

Laminar flow: Friction of the blood elements against the vessel wall causes blood to flow more slowly along the walls of a vessel compared with the velocity in the center of the vessel. The result is a regular variation of flow velocities across a vessel, producing what can be described as a parabolic shape to the flow profile. This type of flow pattern is known as *laminar flow.*

Accelerated flow: When the diameter of a blood vessel narrows, the blood spins can experience an increase in velocity, which can occur in both normal and diseased vessels and can be a source of signal loss in conventional magnetic resonance angiography (MRA) sequences.

Turbulent flow: Turbulent flow can be defined as randomly fluctuating velocities of blood flow within a vessel. Typically, turbulent flow occurs when the velocity passes a critical threshold. The presence of turbulent flow causes a signal loss in conventional MRA sequences.

Vortex-swirling flow: Vortex flow is characterized by a somewhat circular swirling flow pattern. This type of pattern can occur immediately distal to a stenotic area and in normal vessels, particularly at bifurcations or sharp turns. The presence of vortex or swirling flow can contribute to signal loss in conventional MRA sequences.

Triphasic flow: This flow pattern is observed in normal femoral and brachial arteries. During systole, blood flows in the normal antegrade direction. During diastole, however, pressure in the vessel is reduced and the blood actually flows backward (retrograde). The flow again reverses and flows antegrade during late diastole.

Magnetic Resonance Angiography

MRA is the most common magnetic resonance imaging (MRI) application relating to imaging flow. Although the name implies that images of vessels are being produced, with conventional MRA techniques, this is simply not the case. For the most part, MRA acquires images in which the signal intensity is related to flow. The signal produced from flow (e.g., bright or dark) depends on the type of pulse sequence and imaging options selected.

Spin Echo

- Using a spin echo pulse sequence causes flowing blood to appear as a signal void.
- A spin echo pulse sequence uses both 90-degree and 180-degree RF pulses.
- Both pulses are slice-selective.
- For this reason, spins of flowing blood that receive a 90-degree pulse are unlikely to be in the slice to receive the 180-degree pulse.
- To produce an MR signal in a spin echo pulse sequence, spins must "experience" both the 90-degree and 180-degree pulse.
- This effect is more prevalent when the slice is perpendicular to flow.

- MRA sequences that use spin echo are often referred to as *black blood* techniques.

Figure 9-1 illustrates the signal void in the right internal carotid and basilar artery. The right internal carotid is occluded, and high signal can be observed within the vessel.

Gradient Echo

- A gradient echo sequence uses a gradient magnetic field to produce the echo.
- Because the gradient is not slice-selective, but rather, affects all the spins within the area of the coil, flowing blood generally appears bright.
- This effect is further enhanced when short echo times are used, which minimizes the elapsed time between excitation and sampling.
- MRA sequences that use gradient echoes are often referred to as *bright blood* techniques.

Figure 9-2 demonstrates an example of a gradient recalled echo (GRE) sequence acquired on the same patient, as shown in the previous spin echo example. The high signal in the right carotid and basilar artery, normally observed in the presence of flow, should be noted. The absence of flow signal in the left

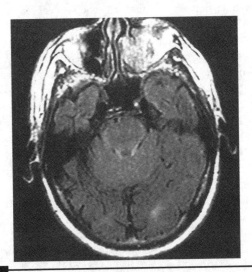

Figure 9-1 An axial FLAIR (spin echo) sequence.

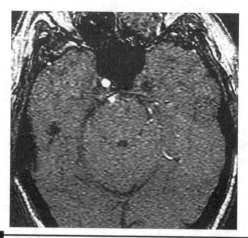

Figure 9-2 A GRE sequence.

internal carotid corresponds with the hyperintense signal in the left internal carotid on the spin echo sequence, consistent with slow or absent flow.

Acquisition and Display

- Most MRA sequences use so-called *bright blood* techniques that employ gradient echo sequences.
- The acquisition parameters (repetition time [TR], echo time [TE], and flip angle) are selected to maximize the saturation effects in background tissues, thereby reducing their MR signal contribution while minimizing the saturation effects on the flowing blood.
- After the images have been acquired, they are often postprocessed to produce images similar in appearance to conventional angiograms.
- Two primary techniques are employed to produce images that are similar to an angiogram: maximum intensity pixel (MIP) for GRE (bright blood) and MIP for spin echo (black blood). Because most sites use GRE sequences for bright blood MRA, the remainder of this text will focus on this technique.
- The source images are "stacked" and the computer draws a ray through the stack at any prescribed angle.

The resulting projection reveals the brightest or darkest pixel along the ray's path.

- To eliminate overlapping vessels, a subvolume can be used for the projections.
- One of the major advantages of MRA is the ability to produce an infinite number of projections or views from a single data set.

The MIP technique, however, has its disadvantages. Because MIP is a projection technique, there is no anatomical information. The image does not represent the vessel but rather, the signal within the vessel. In fact, MIP techniques demonstrate only the brightest pixels. Complex flow patterns can be misrepresented as stenosis or occlusions using the MIP technique. Additionally, anything with a short T1 can appear bright on a GRE-based, time-of-flight (TOF) sequence and can appear as bright as the signal from flowing blood. Examples of these substances include fat and a hemorrhage of a specific age.

REDUCTION OF FLOW ARTIFACTS

Two primary techniques, previously described, are used to reduce flow artifacts: gradient moment nulling (GMN or flow compensation) and spatial presaturation (*sat pulses*, sat bands). GMN is used in MRA sequences to compensate for signal loss from first-order (constant velocity) motion-flow only. Spatial presaturation pulses are used to remove signal from flowing blood, allowing for imaging of flow in one particular direction (e.g., superior-to-inferior or inferior-to-superior).

SIGNAL LOSS IN MRA

Signal loss in MRA can occur for a number of reasons. Recognizing the origins of signal loss and optimizing the pulse sequence and its parameters are important to minimize artifactual signal loss.

- Flow saturation occurs when blood spins are given insufficient time to recover longitudinal magnetization between excitation pulses, which can occur in instances of slow flow or when inappropriate pulse sequence timing parameters (particularly TR and flip angle) are selected.

- Complex flow patterns (such as the patterns mentioned at the beginning of this chapter) are not easily compensated for, which often results in signal loss in an MRA sequence.

- First-order GMN (first-order flow compensation) cannot compensate for accelerated flow, turbulent flow, triphasic flow, or vortex flow.

- The amount of motion between excitation and sampling increases as the TE increases. Short TE times are therefore important in MRA sequences.

- The chance that multidirectional flow or various velocities of flow will exist within a single voxel is increased as the voxel volume is increased.

- Additionally, magnetic susceptibility is directly proportional to both TE and voxel volume. The possibility of signal loss from magnetic susceptibility artifacts is increased as voxel volume is increased.

Two-Dimensional and Three-Dimensional Time-of-Flight

The two basic types of MRA pulse sequences are TOF and phase contrast (PC). Both sequences can be acquired as a two-dimensional (2-D) or three-dimensional (3-D) acquisition. TOF techniques rely on flow-related enhancement to distinguish moving spins from stationary spins.

- In most 2-D TOF MRA acquisitions, the images are acquired sequentially (i.e., the images are acquired and reconstructed one slice at a time).

- In this type of acquisition, the total scan time is equal to the TR times the number of phase encodings times the number of signal averages (NSA) times the number of slices.

- TR times for 2-D TOF sequences are generally short (25 to 50 msec), and the flip angle is generally 45 to 70 degrees. TE times are typically set to be as short as the hardware and/or software will allow.

- When using the TR and flip angles as described with a sequential slice acquisition, the signal from the background tissue is greatly reduced because of saturation.

■ Flowing blood appears bright because unsaturated, fully magnetized blood flows into the slice replacing blood that has received RF pulses.

■ The signal intensity of flow depends on its velocity, the TR, and flip angle.

■ For a given TR and flip angle, the higher the velocity of flowing blood, the greater the MR signal up to the point the spins are fully replaced between TR periods.

■ The lower the velocity, the more RF pulses blood spins receive while in the imaging slice and thus the less intense the MR signal.

■ To image slower velocities, the TR can be reduced or the flip angle can be reduced (saturation reduced).

■ However, when the saturation of slower flowing spins is reduced, the surrounding tissue will be less saturated as well, which can produce less contrast between the stationary tissue and flowing bloods.

■ In general, 2-D TOF techniques work well for vessels with slow to moderate flow velocities.

SIGNAL LOSS WITH TWO-DIMENSIONAL TIME-OF-FLIGHT

■ Flow-related enhancement (FRE) is maximized when the direction of blood flow is perpendicular to the imaging slice.

■ When the vessel turns and the flow is *in-plane* (i.e. parallel with the imaging slice), the spins receive additional RF pulses and thus experience increased saturation. This increase in saturation leads to a reduced signal from flowing spins.

■ Thin slices not only provide for high spatial resolution, but also improve FRE by reducing the time blood spins "spend" in an imaging slice. In most instances, 2-D TOF slices range between 1.5 and 2.0 mm.

■ Thin 2-D slices require high gradient amplitudes for slice selection.

■ Generally, reducing the slice thickness in a 2-D acquisition results in longer echo times and thus increases the likelihood of artifactual signal loss.

- Vessels can often reverse directions, causing the blood to flow back into the imaging slice, which again causes an increase in flow saturation and a reduction in MR signal.
- In the popliteal artery, the normal blood flow pattern is termed *triphasic*. Triphasic flow is characterized by the rapid acceleration of the spins as a result of the systolic contraction of the heart. The arterial blood then flows backwards (superior) during diastole, followed by inferior flow.
- Acquiring the 2-D TOF sequence with cardiac gating or triggering can greatly reduce the phase ghosting observed in the popliteal artery. However, the use of cardiac gating or triggering can often increase the overall scan time and may not be widely available.
- GMN does not compensate for complex flow patterns such as triphasic flow.

Figure 9-3 demonstrates an example of an axial 2-D TOF sequence through the region of the popliteal artery. The signal ghosting from normal triphasic flow is observed on the patient's right side. The left popliteal artery, however, is artifact-free. In this case, the patient has a segmental occlusion on the left, resulting in a loss of the normal triphasic flow pattern.

Three-Dimensional Time-of-Flight

- As the name implies, 3-D TOF techniques acquire data as a 3-D data set.

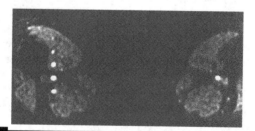

Figure 9-3 An axial 2-D TOF sequence through the region of the popliteal artery.

- The primary advantages of any 3-D acquisition over a 2-D acquisition are improved signal-to-noise ratio (SNR), smaller voxel volumes (improved spatial resolution), and shorter TE.

- The shorter TE and smaller voxel volumes make 3-D TOF more desirable for imaging smaller vessels and less susceptible to signal loss compared with larger voxels and longer TE characteristic of 2-D TOF techniques.

- The primary disadvantage to a 3-D MRA acquisition is its relative insensitivity to slow flow.

- In a 3-D sequence, blood flows through an imaging volume rather than a thin slice.

- As with 2-D TOF, acquiring the data set such that blood flow is perpendicular to the slice direction will optimize FRE.

- However, since a volume (rather than a thin slice) of data is excited, blood spins are in the imaging volume longer and are therefore more prone to saturation.

- For this reason, lower flip angles are used with 3-D TOF sequences compared with 2-D TOF sequences.

- In any event, 3-D TOF acquisitions are less sensitive to slow flow compared with 2-D TOF sequences.

- Because of the lower flip angles used in 3-D TOF acquisitions, the signal from background tissue is not as suppressed compared with 2-D TOF acquisitions.

- To reduce the signal from background tissue, magnetization transfer is a commonly used option.

Magnetization transfer (MT) uses an additional RF pulse applied off-frequency from water.

The MT pulse excites hydrogen protons that are associated with macromolecules such as proteins.

These protons "transfer" some of their magnetization to the water protons, thereby reducing some of their signal. Using MT, gray matter and white matter exhibit a 30% to 40% reduction in MR signal.

Figure 9-4 demonstrates an example of a 3-D TOF sequence acquired with MT. The excellent visualization of the more distal vessels from the improved contrast can be seen.

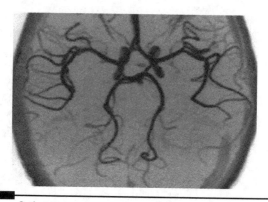

Figure 9-4 A 3-D TOF sequence acquired with magnetization transfer.

Signal Loss with Three-Dimensional Time-of-Flight

- The primary reason for signal loss observed in 3-D TOF MRA is slow flow saturation.
- This effect can be somewhat compensated for by increasing the TR or reducing the flip angle.
- The sequence can be acquired after the intravenous administration of gadolinium, but the normal enhancement patterns of various intracranial structure often reduce the contrast between the blood flow and background tissue.
- Other means of overcoming slow flow saturation include *ramped flip angle* and *multislab* acquisitions.
- In a ramped flip angle acquisition, the flip angle is varied over the imaging voxel in the direction of blood flow (e.g., inferior-to-superior in an axial 3-D TOF study of the circle of Willis).
- For example, if the prescribed flip angle is 30 degrees, then the flip angle in the inferior portion of the imaging slab might be 20 degrees (30 degrees in the middle and 40 degrees at the top).
- Multislab techniques combine the best of 2-D and 3-D acquisitions. Increasing the number of slabs increases the coverage. Saturation is overcome by the use of small slabs.

- The major disadvantage to multislab acquisitions includes longer examination times required for the increased coverage.
- Patient motion can present a problem. When the patient moves between slabs, misregistration can be observed in the MIP images.

PHASE CONTRAST TECHNIQUES

- Phase contrast (PC) techniques rely on velocity-induced phase shifts to differentiate stationary spins from flowing spins.
- A major characteristic of PC images is the complete suppression of background tissue.
- Because of the way PC acquisitions are flow-encoded, they can be used to produce images that are sensitized for either slow flow or fast flow.
- Depending on the type of reconstruction methods used, information regarding the direction of the flow can be attained.
- With additional processing software, using PC to calculate flow velocities is also possible.

Flow Encoding

- Exposure to a gradient magnetic field causes spins along the axis of the gradient field to gain or loose phase, based on their position along the gradient.
- For stationary spins, the amount of phase gained or lost will depend on their position along the gradient, the gradient amplitude, polarity, and the amount of time the gradient field is applied.
- For flowing spins, the amount of phase gained or lost will depend not only on the gradient amplitude, polarity, and duration, but also on the velocity of the flowing spins.
- In a PC acquisition, a toggled pair of bipolar gradients is used for flow encoding (Figure 9-5).
- The reconstruction "looks at" the phase shift and assigns a pixel intensity relative to the amount of phase shift.

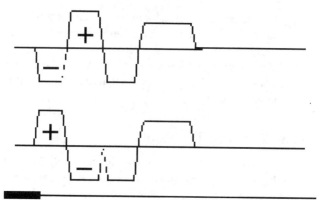

Figure 9-5 In a PC acquisition, a toggled pair of bipolar gradients is used for flow encoding.

- Stationary spins will have a zero net phase shift and thus be subtracted from the final image.
- Flowing spins, however, will have a phase accumulation and thus will be observed on the image.
- The signal intensity displayed will be based on the amount of phase accumulation, which is directly related to the velocity of the spins.
- As mentioned, the flow encoding gradients are applied as a toggled pair.
- With the second encoding, the gradient polarity is reversed.
- The two acquisitions are then subtracted to increase visualization of flow within the vessels.
- The two main methods of subtraction are complex difference and phase difference.
- Complex difference "looks at" the amount of phase shift and displays a positive pixel value of any flow with a velocity greater than zero. The complex difference subtraction method is commonly used with thick slab acquisitions.
- Phase difference "looks at" the angle (ϕ) between the two phase shifts produced by the toggled gradient pair and displays flow direction by pixel sign (black or white).

Velocity Encoding

- The operator can select the velocity sensitivity of a PC acquisition. That is, the operator can choose to make the flow encoding sensitive to slow or fast flow velocities.
- The parameter is referred to as the velocity encoding (VENC).
- VENC determines the amplitude and duration of the flow encoding gradients.
- Low values of VENC highlight slower flow and use stronger flow encoding gradients.
- High values of VENC highlight faster flow and use weaker flow encoding gradients.
- For example, if a VENC of 40 cm/sec is selected, then the flow encoding gradients will be applied such that spins flowing at 40 cm/sec will experience maximal phase shift (180 degrees).
- With the complex difference subtraction, the reconstruction technique cannot differentiate between spins flowing faster than the VENC value and the spins flowing slower than the VENC value. Both values will be reconstructed with lower signal.
- When using phase difference subtraction, spins flowing faster than the VENC value have phase shifts of spins flowing in the opposite direction and are displayed as such.
- These reconstruction errors are known as aliasing.
- One way to consider the VENC is to say that it represents the fastest velocity that can be displayed without aliasing.

In summary, the major advantages of phase contrast include:

- Complete suppression of background (nonflowing) spins.
- The ability to image slow or fast flow.
- The ability to acquire information relating to flow direction.

Index

Spin density, 23
Spin echo inversion sequence, 34
Spin echo pulse sequences, 26-27
  chemical shift and, 68
  fast; see Fast spin echo sequences
  hemorrhage and, 69
  inversion recovery and, 28
  magnetic resonance angiography and, 82-83
  magnetic susceptibility and, 68
  presaturation pulses and, 71
  slice selection and, 40
Spin excess, 14
Spin states, 13-14
Spine, 7, 31
Spin-lattice relaxation, 24
Spin-spin relaxation, 21, 24
Spoiled GRE, 33-34
Spoiling, 34
Static magnetic field, 1, 5
Stationary spins, 91-92
Steady state GRE, 33-34
Stenosis, 85
STIR; see Short T1 recovery sequences
Stroke, 35
Superconductive magnets, 3-4
Superconductivity, 3
Surface coils, 2, 6-7, 55, 61
Systole, 82, 88

T

256-frequency encoding, 40-41
T1 relaxation, 21, 24
T1 relaxation time, image contrast and, 29-30
T1 time, 21
T1 weighting, 30, 36
  flip angle and, 32
  inversion recovery sequences and, 34
T2 decay, 24
T2 relaxation, 21, 23-24
T2 relaxation times, image contrast and, 28-29
T2 weighting, 28-29, 30-32
T2*, 21, 26, 32, 33
Target TE, 49

Tau, 27
TE; see Time to echo
Temperature, 2, 24
Temporomandibular joint, 7
Tesla, 12-13
Thermal equilibrium, 14, 15
Three-dimensional acquisitions, 9, 61-62, 70
Three-dimensional time-of-flight, 86-87, 88-91
TI; see Time of inversion
Time of inversion, 28, 34
Time to echo
  in- and out-of-phase, 68
  image contrast and, 28-29, 30-31
  magnet susceptibility and, 69-70
  magnetic resonance angiography and, 84, 86
  signal-to-noise ratio and, 55
  spin echo sequences and, 26-27, 28
  three-dimensional time-of-flight and, 89
  two-dimensional time-of-flight and, 86-87
Timing parameters, signal-to-noise ratio and, 55-56
Tissue characteristics, 23-24
TR; see Repetition time
T/R coil, 6
Transmit-and-receive coil, 6
Transverse magnetization, 17, 23-24
Triphasic flow, 82, 86, 88
Truncation artifact, 78
Turbo spin echo, 48
Turbulent flow, 81-82, 86
Two-dimensional acquisitions, 44, 61
Two-dimensional time-of-flight, 86-88

U

U. S. Food and Drug Administration, 4

V

Velocity, 87
Velocity encoding, 93